I0665070

The Shakespeare Drug

The Shakespeare Drug

K. Scot Macdonald

Kerrera House Press

Copyright © 2012 by K. Scot Macdonald

All rights reserved. No part of this publication may be reproduced, transmitted in any form or by any means, graphic, electronic or mechanical, including photo-copying, recording, taping or by any information storage retrieval system, without the permission in writing from the publisher.

The characters, institutions and events in this novel are creations of the author's imagination. Any likeness to persons, institutions or events, living or dead, past or present, is purely coincidental.

Macdonald, K. Scot.
The Shakespeare Drug/K. Scot Macdonald—1st Edition
p.   cm.
ISBN 978-0-9859650-0-6

Kerrera House Press
Culver City, CA
www.KerreraHousePress.com

First Printing: 2012
Printed in the United States of America

10 9 8 7 6 5 4 3 2 1

For Dad,

Dreams do come true.

I contain multitudes.

—Walt Whitman, "Song of Myself," 1855

November

Julie Stein concentrated on delicately using a sphenoid punch to cut a hole through the roof of Tom Morris' optic canal, taking extreme care to avoid cutting into either the ethmoid or sphenoid sinus. She stared at the image on a monitor transmitted via a snake-like endoscope from inside the patient's skull. The light-gray tumor had spread from the pituitary gland at the base of the brain and wrapped itself around Mr. Morris' optic nerve. The sight of the location and size of the tumor confirmed her diagnosis of why the geriatric patient's field of vision had shrunk to the size of a fist at arm's length.

Wiggling her jaw and rolling her shoulders to ease the tension in them, Julie fumed at the thought of Andrew Baxter pushing her to perform the procedure.

"You will do it," Baxter pronounced the day before.

"I would really prefer not to," Julie said, well aware that she was speaking to the Chair of Neurosurgery, Director of the Short-Lo Neurosurgical Institute and holder of the Micheal and Janette

O'Keeffe Chair in Neurosciences at Mount Hermon Medical Center, not to mention her boss.

"You will." Baxter's pale blue eyes locked on her dark eyes with a chilling intensity.

"Mr. Morris is 82 years old," Julie said, her voice calm, yet firm. Baxter had hired her and she respected, even envied him, but there was no way she would just give in. She knew she was right—or at least as certain as you could ever be in medicine. "The risk of the procedure far outweighs any possible foreseeable benefit."

The tension in Julie's jaws and shoulders returned as she recalled squaring off in Baxter's corner office with its expansive views across West Los Angeles, which the previous morning had been unimpaired by even a particle of smog. One wall of the office was covered with Baxter's bachelors of science, masters of business administration and medical degrees surrounded by framed medical journal covers from *The Lancet, New England Journal of Medicine, Journal of Neurosurgery* and *Stroke* featuring articles by researchers from the laboratory he directed. One benefit of being director was that regardless of his level of input, Baxter's name went on every article any researcher in the laboratory published. Along the low, metal window sills perched pictures of Baxter and his family sailing the Caribbean, climbing—really a strenuous hike from what Julie had heard—Mount Kilimanjaro, and taking a hot-air balloon ride over Angkor Wat in Kampuchea. There were also photos of Baxter with a couple of U.S. presidents, the Prime Minister of Canada, and enough celebrities to cast a big-budget movie.

"He needs the surgery," Baxter insisted. "You said he's beginning to experience seizures."

"Well managed with anti-seizure medication."

"He's going blind."

"Better blind than dead on the table."

At forty-seven, Baxter was at the height of his profession and, Julie knew, he was far from used to being told no. He pursed his thin lips, blew air out of his nostrils and tried another tack. "You've gone over all the risks with him?"

"Yes."

"He's competent to understand those risks?"

"Yes," Julie admitted grudgingly, already knowing where this was headed.

"Then perform the procedure."

"I won't."

Baxter sighed, rocked in his leather chair and ran a well-scrubbed hand through his short, black, gray-streaked hair. "What does his family say?"

"His wife is…worried about the risks."

Baxter sensed Julie's hesitancy. "But?"

"She supports his decision, as do his children."

"Perform the procedure."

"No." Julie knew her job might be at stake, but the more Baxter pressed, the more determined she became to refuse. She had no intention of gaining a reputation as a pushover. It was already tough enough being one of only about 150 female neurosurgeons out of 3,600 such specialists in the country.

"Julie, please," Baxter said, leaning in supplication across his oak desk with the green baize inset. "I would do it myself but I have to be on a plane to Washington in two hours for the Congressional hearings on stem cell research tomorrow." He glanced at his leather-strapped watch to emphasize the point.

"Severn can do it. He's never busy."

Baxter pursed his lips, narrowed his eyes and tilted his head to the side in shocked disbelief. "Julie, you're the finest surgeon for pituitary tumors we have—anyone has—in the country, if not the world. Tom Morris will have the procedure. If you don't do it, he'll find someone else to do it and the risk will be higher. It's your choice, but I'd hate to have to live with it if he goes somewhere else, has the procedure and goes blind or worse, dies."

"Dafoe can do it. He's almost as good as I am." No neurosurgeon would ever admit that another was 'as good' as they were.

"He wants you."

"Tell him I had an emergency and couldn't do it."

Blanching at the effrontery of such a suggestion, Baxter exclaimed, "I'm not going to lie to Tom Morris."

"A white lie."

"Not if something goes wrong."

"Then you agree," Julie said, pouncing. "It's risky."

"Having your appendix out is risky," Baxter said with a dismissive wave of his hand, his voice rising as he sought to control his temper.

"If he wants to have it done, he can go somewhere else."

"Somewhere else?" Baxter's eyes widened. "Do you know how much he's given to this hospital over the past 20 years? The Morris Cancer Institute, the Morris Fellowship Program, and go out and read the name on the research building some time—all eight stories of it."

Julie shook her head, no.

"He's a famous man, Julie," Baxter said, smiling that beckoning, warm smile that convinced bottom-line business people and jaded movie stars to hand over millions of dollars every year to support his department and its research efforts. "Whoever operates on him will be famous."

"No."

"More cases, more prestige, more research funding." Baxter paused, then added, "more money for you. This could make the career I've always thought you could have."

"I don't want to start doing surgeries based on their PR value."

"That's not what I meant and you know it." Baxter clenched his straight, white teeth and then sighed to release his mounting frustration. He picked up a gold mechanical pencil and tapped it on the beveled edge of his desk. Staring Julie straight in the eye, he pleaded while keeping a dignified tone, "For the hospital, Julie, for Mr. Morris and his family, for me, for you, please do it."

Julie paused. Baxter had hired her. She owed him, not a lot—three other medical centers had wanted her talents in their ORs and research labs—but she did owe him something. Putting her relationship with Baxter in the scales against her medical judgment, she reached a decision. "'I will prescribe regimens for the good of my patients according to my ability and my judgment, and never do harm to anyone.'"

"Don't quote the Hippocratic oath to me," Baxter commanded, his voice rising to a crescendo. His voice bordering on a yell, he ordered, "He wants the procedure done and you will do it."

"I won't," Julie said, keeping her voice calm. She would never give anyone the chance to dismiss her as 'just another emotional woman.'

"He knows the risks, he's competent to understand them and he wants you to do the surgery. His wife and family want it done. This hospital wants you to do it. I want you to do it, so do it."

Julie was on the verge of saying that the state medical board would be interested in hearing about a medical director ordering a surgeon to perform a surgery the surgeon believed was medically inappropriate when Baxter added, lowering his voice, "The bottom line is, he wants it done, so please do it."

"He wants it done so he can see to play golf."

"I don't care if he wants it done so he can use up his health-insurance deductible," Baxter said, losing his patience. "You will do what your patient wants, for God's sake."

"It's not in his best interest."

"Who are you to judge that?"

"I'm his doctor."

"You're his surgeon. What does his PCP say?"

Julie flicked a piece of non-existent lint from her black slacks.

Baxter flipped through a thick file on his desk. Finding the name of Morris' primary care physician, he asked, "What does O'Neill say?"

Julie hesitated, tapped her index finger on her thigh—the thought flashing through her mind that she should run six miles the next morning or she would never be in shape in time for the LA Marathon—and said, "He recommends the procedure." Her eyes flashed up to meet Baxter's before he could pounce. "He's not a surgeon. He doesn't know the risks for an 82 year old."

"He knows his patient." Baxter tossed the gold pencil on his desk and, leaning back said, "What do you put the mortality risk at?"

"Twenty percent."

"I wouldn't think it's near that high."

"You don't know the patient." Before Baxter could respond, Julie continued, "High blood pressure, arrhythmia a few years ago, high cholesterol, osteoporosis, asthma, hypothyroidism from the tumor, and he's allergic to enough drugs to fill two typed pages—and that's just the ones we know of."

Baxter made a point of appearing to consider the information. "Closer to five percent, I would think. If you use Collingwood for anesthesia, it should be even lower, less than one percent."

"The risk of a stroke is high. Might not kill him, but he'll never play golf again."

"He'll never play golf again without the procedure. He'll go blind."

Julie waited a moment, pushed her shoulder-length, brown hair behind her ears and said, "No."

Baxter pushed his oxblood leather chair back on its soundless castors, rose and stalked over to glare out a window. It was warm in the office. The sun beat on the windows and the building's air conditioning, while keeping most of the building at a comfortable 70 degrees, failed to attain that temperature in the south-facing offices. After a moment's thought, Baxter turned and asked, "You had a difficult pregnancy with Pete, didn't you?"

Uncertain where this sudden change in direction was going, Julie nodded cautiously.

"How bad was it?"

"I could have died," Julie admitted, remembering and beginning to see Baxter's line of thought, yet not believing he would use such a vile tactic.

"You were willing to die for your baby."

'Bastard,' she thought, but said, "It's different."

"How?"

"Golf's not a baby."

"People value different things."

"Everyone values their children more than some game—more than anything."

Baxter failed to convince her. Mr. Morris succeeded, but only after an hour and a half conversation. A born salesman, Mr. Morris was a persuasive man. More importantly, he knew the risks and, as Baxter had pointed out, Mr. Morris had the money and connections to go anywhere to have the procedure done. Julie knew she had the best chance of making the operation a success, so she better be the one to do it.

Yesterday Julie had thought the procedure would be risky. Now able to see inside Mr. Morris's skull base, she realized it was even more risky than she had thought. Usually pituitary tumors put pressure on the optic nerve, but don't grow around the nerve itself. In fact, few pituitary tumors spread at all. Mr. Morris was just one of the unlucky few. Removing a tumor that was involved with the optic nerve carried a high risk of loss of vision in the affected eye. Mr. Morris would be lucky to come out of the procedure with his vision intact. The question of whether you could play golf with one eye crossed Julie's mind.

Banishing such thoughts, she locked her eyes on the shadowy, moving images on the 24-inch monitor. Just after cutting into Mr. Morris's skull base, she had mapped the tumor using the intraoperative MRI, which delineated the exact location of the tumor mass. The tumor could shift when the skull was opened, so the intraoperative MRI provided a more accurate location for the tumor than an MRI taken before surgery could provide.

Julie scraped globs of tumor cells from the nerve, which was half the width of a pencil, nestled within the narrow confines of the optic canal. The pale tumor cells were barely discernable against the grayish healthy brain cells.

"You have to be extremely careful," Julie told the attentive resident assisting her. "The optic nerve can't regenerate, so make certain you only scrape off tumor cells; no healthy cells."

It was like trying to pick a line of soggy Cheerios out of a bowl of cold porridge, all while manipulating surgical instruments up through the patient's sinus cavity via their nose. Blood obscured the image on the monitor from the endoscope faster than the suction cleared it.

"Is the suction clogged?" Julie asked the resident as she used a drill with her blue-gloved right hand to widen the hole in the optic canal. She needed greater access to resect more of the tumor. The pungent smell of burning bone assaulted her nostrils even through her mask.

Over the high-pitched whirr of the drill, the phone on the off-white wall of the OR rang. A nurse answered it.

The resident inspected the clear tube that ran from the suction-irrigation device in Julie's non-dominant left hand to the floor where it connected to a red-lidded transparent container containing a quarter inch of blood. "Seems to be working."

"It's weak," Julie said. "I'm getting some heat from the drilling. I don't want to damage the optic nerve or he'll never see his house again, let alone a golf ball."

"Saline transfers the heat away from the optic nerve?" the resident half-asked.

"If it's flowing fast enough." Julie jiggled the suction ever so slightly. "It's working better now. Might have been clogged with bone chips."

"Dr. Stein," the nurse who had answered the phone called, "the wife of one of your research subjects is waiting to see you at clinic."

"I don't have any appointments today," Julie said as she kept her concentration on the monitor, scraping a few more tumor cells off the nerve, although her voice betrayed that she might be mistaken about her appointment schedule.

"Sandy says she just showed up; said it's an emergency."

"Then call 9-1-1," Julie said, keeping her attention on the difficult procedure she was performing.

"She said it wasn't that kind of emergency; something to do with body and soul, and keeping them together."

"Call the rabbi then."

The nurses and techs laughed.

"Sandy said she most definitely has to see you."

"This could take another hour," Julie warned, making sure to keep any hint of frustration out of her voice.

The nurse conveyed the information. "She says she'll wait."

Julie wondered what the woman could want. Reminded of the outside world, Julie glanced up at the clock. "Call Mr. Morris's wife and tell her everything's going fine. It's just taking a little longer than expected. Tell her he's doing great."

Julie returned to her painstaking scraping. With its mass of nerves, tendons and eloquent parts of the brain nearby, the skull base was one of the most complex parts of the body in which to operate.

"You follow the nerve into the tumor as you resect the tumor piecemeal," she told the resident, who nodded as he alternated between watching the monitor and Julie's hands as she delicately manipulated the surgical instruments.

"Make sure the tumor hasn't spread into the cavernous sinus." Without turning Julie asked the anesthesiologist, Collingwood, huddled before a bank of gauges, cylinders and monitors near the unconscious patient's head, "How's he doing?"

"Stable and well," the middle-aged Collingwood reported. Even so, the veteran, black anesthesiologist closely monitored his patient's vital signs. Laid out on a blue sterile towel beside him were syringes with various drugs that would be required if any one of a multitude of things went wrong. Beside them sat Collingwood's laptop, which was connected to speakers perched atop his wheeled console.

"Who are we listening to today?" Julie asked, still scraping tumor cells, but trying to stay relaxed enough to finely control her hand movements. Tension could make her hands cramp and reduce her fine-motor control.

"Rita MacNeil," Collingwood replied.

A nurse asked, "Who?"

"Scots-Canadian country and folk singer from Big Pond, Nova Scotia," Collingwood reported, his jolly, baritone voice filling the OR.

"No wonder I'd never heard of her," the nurse said.

Julie said, "I've never even heard of Big Pond."

Forty-five minutes later, Julie withdrew the endoscope, her instruments and the suction-irrigation device from Mr. Morris's skull. Drained, yet full of adrenaline after the challenging procedure, she was relieved it had gone so well. The laboratory would soon report whether the tumor cells were cancerous, yet she already suspected that Mr. Morris had the bad luck to have a rare cancerous pituitary tumor. In medicine, rarity was a bad thing. The best thing to have was a common condition that doctors had a great deal of experience diagnosing and treating.

If the tumor was cancerous, an MRI would show whether Julie had achieved the desired 99.9 percent resection. It sounded like an impossible goal, but a tumor might contain 10 billion cancer cells. If a surgeon removed 90 percent of the tumor, the patient would still be host to a billion tumor cells. Those cells would multiply and spread, requiring another surgery—if the patient survived long enough. If Julie achieved a 99.9 percent resection, chemotherapy and radiation should kill the remaining cancer cells.

"Let's make sure the optic nerve and oculomotor nerves are decompressed," Julie said, looking through the slit between her mask and her surgical cap at the resident, "then we'll take another MRI and see how we did."

Having checked the nerves, Julie stood aside and wiggled her toes in her clogs to warm them in the cold OR. Two techs trundled the intraoperative MRI out of its closet. The imaging machine resembled two thick, blue garbage can lids on their sides two feet apart attached to a metal box the size of a three-drawer filing cabinet. The techs rolled the machine into position so that Mr. Morris' head was between the "lids." The "lids" were actually powerful magnets. To avoid having the magnets drain their batteries and wipe their memories clean, everyone placed their watches, cell phones, pagers, Collingwood's laptop, and all other pieces of electronic equipment in a lead-lined cabinet built into the wall. Two techs rolled the monitor on its stand and other electronic equipment out of the OR. A second MR image was taken in the now silent OR.

Before the introduction of the intraoperative MRI, a scan could not be taken until after the patient was rolled out of the OR. If it was discovered that more than .1 percent of the tumor remained, the patient would have to return for another procedure. With the intraoperative MRI, the surgeon could immediately go back in to resect any discernable tumor spotted on the MRI image without having to perform another complete operation.

A few minutes later Julie and the resident peered at the scan on a wall monitor. An extra pair of eyes never hurt in trying to see any suspicious white or fuzzy objects. The resident asked, "See anything?"

*Only when he no longer knows what he is
doing does the painter do good things.*

—Edgar Degas, French artist, 1834-1917

"My dear, Julie, how are you?" Rick Severn, a thrice-divorced neurosurgeon in his late forties asked, pausing to chat on the covered pedestrian bridge between the hospital and the Medical Office Towers. With short black hair, Severn had the rugged good looks of a cigarette-ad cowboy and a body honed by Ironman competitions encased in a pin-striped suit. The triathlons took the place of surgery for him since he rarely operated. Everyone knew that he loathed his ex-wives and by not operating he kept his income at the level of a color-blind house painter. Severn's divorce attorney had thrice argued that a surgeon's income varied year to year and judges had thrice foolishly set alimony as a percentage of Severn's income. By rarely operating Severn ensured that his detested ex-wives received miniscule alimony payments.

"Just resected a pituitary tumor," Julie replied. She could smell his cologne, which brought thoughts of a warm, soothing bath to her tired legs, back and arms after the long procedure. "Heavily involved with the optic nerve. Cancerous."

"Rare, but challenging," Severn said, a trace of longing in his voice. "How'd it go?"

"Ninety-nine point nine percent resection."

"If I ever need a piece of my pituitary removed, you'll be the first person I call," Severn proclaimed heartily.

"Better not, I may remove your frontal lobe."

"What have I done to deserve such a dire threat?" Severn asked, recoiling in mock fear.

"You treated Anthony De Stirling and didn't even introduce me."

"Emergency coiling of an AVM. In and out the same evening; drive-through neurosurgery."

"It was Anthony De Stirling."

"He's just a writer. We've treated movie stars, pro athletes and titans of industry. What's the big deal?"

"'Just a writer'? He's written 23 novels, won the Pulitzer twice, four National Book Awards and there's talk he's being considered for a Nobel."

"Okay, then just a good writer," Severn said with a sardonic grin.

"If you ever treat any other writers, however you rate them, please promise to let me know."

"Of course. If I'd known you were infatuated with writers, I would have introduced you to De Stirling. By the way, I do some writing on the side…" His voice trailed off as he raised an eyebrow and looked down at her with a comically exaggerated leer.

"Publish a few novels, then maybe I'll consider going out with you."

"Well, if that's the case, I'm off to lunch at Morton's."

"With a pretty pharma rep?" Julie asked with a mischievous grin.

Chuckling, Severn corrected Julie, "A pretty medical-device rep."

Given that he rarely operated and rarely saw patients, Severn spent his ample spare time, besides training for triathlons, being wined and dined by every pharmaceutical company and medical device representative in Los Angeles. Such reps were usually pretty, single young women, often ex-nurses. The companies were more than willing to pay for expensive lunches and dinners in exchange for Severn's good word on the many committees he served on, again given his ample spare time.

Checking his black, aquatic watch, Severn said, "Sorry, must go."

"Mustn't keep a pretty girl waiting."

"Perish the thought," Severn called over his shoulder with a genial wave as he strode toward the hospital. "I'd never let you wait a millionth of a second, my dear."

Julie took the stairs two at a time up to her office in the Medical Office Towers. As she hurried past her assistant's cubicle, Sandy said, "Mail," and handed Julie a stack of opened envelopes. The blonde, just-noticeably-overweight assistant called after Julie, "Mrs. Croft is waiting in Clinic 6 and Hsu is waiting for you over at the lab."

Julie nodded. She sped into her office as she leafed through the mail. On top, Sandy had placed a request to guest lecture on skull-base surgery at the University of Chicago, a letter of acceptance from *The Lancet* for a paper Julie had first-authored on the use of a drug cocktail to treat memory deficits related to Alzheimer's disease, and a letter from a drug company asking if she would serve as an outside reviewer on one of their drug studies for the treatment of Lewy Body Dementia. Sandy had highlighted with a pink marker that the review would take place in Geneva with five-star accommodations, all expenses paid; not that any of that would affect the conclusions of any of the doctors who attended.

Julie's office was on the eighth floor overlooking a narrow plaza with ornamental trees in terra cotta planters between it and the hospital's south tower. Twice while sitting at her desk Julie had seen people jump: one an AIDS patient who, before there was effective treatment for the disease, had somehow reached the roof of the nine story South Tower and leapt off; the other a young woman who had taken off her pink shoes and, laying her purse on top of them, had climbed onto the broad ledge along the edge of the plaza and stepped off to fall three stories to the loading dock below. The AIDS patient died; the young woman, whom Julie treated as neurosurgeon on call, survived.

Julie pushed her door closed with her clogged foot—clogs were far more comfortable to wear in the OR than closed shoes; you could slip your foot out and wiggle each one in turn while you stood operating—and grabbed a white lab coat off the wood hanger behind the door. "Julie Stein, MD, PhD, Department of Neurosurgery" was stitched in blue lettering over the left breast. As she slipped the coat on and slid out of her clogs and into a pair of basic, black slip-ons, she dropped the mail on her cherry desk and reluctantly pulled an envelope out of the stack that had caught her eye. The letterhead bore a stylized range of green mountains and the words, "Appalachian Literary Journal. Established 1896."

Bowing to the inevitable, Julie slid out the letter and skimmed it: "regret to inform you," "given the volume of submissions," and "We wish you the best of luck in placing your short story in another more suitable publication."

Pursing her lips and letting out a sigh, she stepped past her floor-to-ceiling bookcases. On the top shelves were neurosurgical texts and journals. The lower less-visible shelves held English 19th Century novels, a few modern novels and a row of writing books. She stopped at a wood filing cabinet, which contained two drawers of medical articles she was writing or had published, and two drawers of unpublished novels and short stories. She kept one copy of each at home and one at the hospital. That way if her house burned down she would still have copies. She pulled the top drawer out and her long, unadorned fingers found a two-inch thick file labeled in heavy black ink: Rejections. She pried it open and slid in the latest result of her literary efforts. This could not continue.

"He painted a wee bit when we were first married, but he soon got that silliness out of his system," Mrs. Croft explained when Julie arrived in clinic exam room 6, her lab coat camouflaging her scrubs. She usually wore a suit or at least a conservative blouse and slacks on days she saw patients, but Mrs. Croft's visit was unexpected.

"But now, Lord above, Dr. Stein, he spends most of the day in his little room in the garage painting and dabbing and making a grand mess." Mrs. Croft was short, gray-haired and shaped like a block of marble with broad, square shoulders and a square head to match. Her brown dress, black square-toed shoes and a brown wool coat did nothing to dispel Julie's notion that she was a colorless individual. "You'd think his life depended on it," Mrs. Croft rambled on. "Behind his back I have to keep throwing out paintings or finding people to give them to or there wouldn't be any room left in the whole place for us to live, let alone for my tea cup collection."

"I'm glad he's still active, Mrs. Croft," Julie said, wondering where this was leading.

"Active?" the gray-haired lady asked, aghast, leaning forward in the clinic room's hard plastic chair, which squeaked. "Last month he couldn't figure out what a light bulb was for when I asked him to change the one in the hall, and now he mixes paints until the fumes seep into the house even from the garage, hammers canvases onto frames at all hours and paints every waking hour, talking about the influence of light on the banana tree in the backyard and which perspective is best to paint flowers, as if I'd have the foggiest notion or care about any such silliness."

"So you'd say the new drug combination is having a positive effect on Mr. Croft?"

"I don't know about positive; he's certainly changed."

Julie hoped the positive change would be supported by her testing. "Well, thank you for coming in," she said as she moved toward the door. She had her research assistant to see, four procedure dictations to do, a paper to review for *Pediatric Neurosurgery*, and she had to call the medical directors of three insurance companies to get approvals for various imaging studies that had been rejected for three of her patients. The medical directors always agreed to the scans once she explained the reasoning behind their necessity, but the calls took valuable time out of her day during which she could have been seeing patients, operating or conducting research. She also had a football game to attend that night.

"I know you cover the cost of the drugs and testing and such, Dr. Stein," Mrs. Croft went on, clutching her black handbag as she rose from her chair, but remaining where she stood. "But I wondered if you could see fit to cover the cost of some of his art supplies. He's painting us out of house and home. I haven't had any money to buy so much as a saucer in months."

"I am sorry, but there's no money in the trial budget for art supplies." Julie opened the door to reveal the bare, pale blue hall that led to the waiting area. "Although we could certainly use some art around here."

If winning isn't everything,
why do they keep score?

—Vince Lombardi, US football coach,
1913-1970

December

"It's second and one on the Santa Maria Spartans' one-yard line."
The radio announcer's staccato voice went out over the airwaves to
tens of thousands of listeners. "Spartans up 17-14. We'll know the
winner of the Los Angeles Division I High School Championship
in just 14 ticks of the game clock."

With the thunder and roar of the 27,000 fans at the Home
Depot Center in Carson, just southwest of downtown Los Angeles deafening him, Pete Tomlinson's intense eyes, stung by sweat,
scanned the Vandals' backfield. Coach had sent in a pass-defense
play. With a cornerback Pete was supposed to double-team one of
the Vandals' elusive wide receivers.

"The Vandals can either try two quick passes or risk a run, gambling they can stop the clock with their final time-out before time
expires.

"Billy Rogers, the Vandals' lanky, junior quarterback, comes up
to the line and starts his count. Rogers glances back at his lone run-

ning back: Kaylor Smith. The top running back in the state, Smith is 6' 2" and 210 pounds with 2,416 yards rushing and 36 touchdowns for the year; a one-man scoring machine."

Pete saw the glance. They're going to run. Coach sent in the wrong play. On impulse, Pete moved up to be ready to slice through the line and into the backfield to tackle Smith before he gained even a yard.

"Tomlinson!" Coach Paukenan screamed at Pete. "Get into position! Outside! Get outside!"

Pete steeled his nerves and ignored his coach. He knew he was right.

"Rogers gives a hard count," the announcer reported to his rapt audience. "No Spartans drawn offside."

His hands twitching with nervous energy, Pete lined up with the narrow gap between the left guard and tackle.

"Hike!"

"The ball's snapped. Rogers takes three steps back and pivots right to throw. His receivers cut into the end zone, blanketed by the Spartans cornerbacks and both safeties."

Pete launched himself into the sliver of a gap.

"Rogers pump fakes. The defensive linemen raise their hands to block a pass. No, wait, with no one open, Rogers hands off to Smith."

Turning sideways, Pete threaded the six-inch slot between the guard and tackle.

"Ball held tight, Smith cuts to the left and bounces along the line, looking for a hole that isn't there. Wait, no, he finds one, but he's rushed right into the arms of the Spartans' middle linebacker, Tomlinson."

Pete felt the impact and then the strength in Smith's legs as the back spun and juked. Smith dug into the turf with his cleats, driving forward to gain every inch he could. For an instant, Pete thought he was going to lose hold of the whirling dervish that was Smith. His muscles screamed and burned from the effort, but then, finally, Pete brought Smith down.

Smith threw the ball into the turf and tried to stand, but Pete hung on to him just that extra few seconds to piss him off.

"You ain't going anywhere," Pete promised Smith, "ever."

"Fuck off, pussy."

"Tomlinson takes down Smith for no gain," the announcer reported. "It's third and goal from the seven. Vandals' time out; their final one. Six seconds left on the game clock."

Having chugged down water from a cute water-girl to counteract the dehydrating effects of the game on such a hot, dry, southern California night, Pete closed his eyes, shrugged his shoulders and shook out his arms and legs. He was ready. He had never felt better.

The cornerback Ogarsky told Pete, "Coach says you do that again, you're benched."

Pete glanced over at his glaring coach. Did he mean ignoring his play call or tackling a running back for a loss?

"Timeout over. The Spartans have substituted a dime formation: four linemen, one linebacker and six defensive backs. Tomlinson is the lone linebacker. Coach Paukenan is betting on a pass.

"Vandals line up showing pass with four wide receivers, two on each side to spread the Spartans' defense, no tight ends and a lone running back: Smith.

"Rogers strides up to center, surveys the defense, checks his receivers and crouches to begin his count.

"Tomlinson rushes up to threaten the right guard, then backs off as Rogers starts the count; a fast count. The center snaps the ball."

Pete cursed, caught backing up just as the play started.

"All the receivers are in motion, bouncing off the defending backs before they cut past them to run their routes in the end zone."

Watching Rogers' eyes, Pete dodged along behind his linemen.

"Rogers looks right, center, back left corner of the end zone. Every receiver covered. Nothing there. Rogers pump fakes and again; still no one free. The Vandals' line is doing a magnificent protection job, but it's starting to crumble. Smith is in motion. With nowhere to throw, Rogers hands Smith the ball."

Pete rounded the left end and surged into the Vandals' backfield. The end got an arm on him. It slowed him just enough to allow Rogers to complete the handoff.

"Rogers throws a rolling block at the onrushing Tomlinson. Smith takes a step forward, sees nothing. He bounces to the left and speeds around the left end of the Spartans line. Not a Spartan near him.

"Hurdling Rogers, Tomlinson streaks across the backfield after Smith. Smith, two steps ahead, drives for the end zone, just three strides away.

"Tomlinson launches himself at Smith. Tomlinson misses Smith—hold it: Tomlinson has Smith's right foot."

Smith's heel kicked Pete in the facemask. Hanging on, his head ringing and vision blurred from the kick, Pete threw himself down onto the chewed-up turf. Smith was still on his left foot, hopping toward the end zone with Pete in tow.

"If Smith falls forward, he'll score and the Vandals win. Tomlinson spins Smith away from the end zone, using Smith's leg as a lever.

"Tomlinson and Smith grapple, each bent on achieving their goal: Tomlinson to bring Smith down; Smith to reach the ball into the end-zone—just out of reach.

"Two Spartans hit Smith. They topple sideways. Smith lands on top of Tomlinson. Tomlinson's arms are still wrapped around Smith's right shoe. Smith reaches as far as he can with the ball toward the goal line. He's done it! Touchdown Vandals! Time has run out! The Vandals are the new Los Angeles City champions!"

"You made eight tackles and caught four passes," Julie Stein said, as she followed her exhausted and devastated son, Pete, into their California bungalow in Santa Maria, West Los Angeles. His dark head was bowed forward, his muscular shoulders sagged and his feet dragged as he shambled into the house. Julie felt his dejection like a black aura engulfing him, sending dark wisps of despair out in every direction.

Pete nodded, his face glum.

"You almost saved the game."

"Almost."

He crawled off to his room. Although he played middle linebacker and tight end, he dreamed only of being a middle linebacker in the NFL. His room's walls were covered with posters of the finest linebackers his favorite team, the Chicago Bears, had ever produced: Bill George, Dick Butkus, Mike Singletary and Brian Urlacher. There was also one center, George Trafton, a Hall of Famer who basically played middle linebacker before the position existed and, her son had told Julie with great relish, once put four opposing players out of commission in the first dozen plays of a 1920 game. Her son's heroes.

Years before Julie had tried to interest Pete in Jewish football stars she found on the Internet; Sid Luckman, Lyle Alzedo and, Julie's favorite, Ron Mix, who was known as the "Intellectual Assassin" for his physical, yet controlled and intelligent play. Mix only garnered two holding penalties in ten years as a left tackle and guard. With no support from Pete's Anglo-Irish father, Julie failed to elicit much interest in Jewish players and Pete stuck with his Chicago linebackers, regardless of religion, race or nickname.

Julie was considering whether to go in and face the daunting task of trying to console Pete, when she noticed the red light on the answering machine in the kitchen blinking.

I've found that prayers work best
when you have big players.

—Knute Rockne, Norwegian-born,
US football coach, 1888-1931

Julie hit the answering machine button and poured herself a glass of water as she rubbed her eyes. With the Santa Anas blowing, her eyes were red and sore from the pollution, pollen and dust the hot, dry winds blew in from the desert across the city to the coast.

"This message is for Pete Tomlinson. This is Dave Hancock, defensive coordinator for the University of Southern California. Just wanted to let you know I was at the game tonight. Sorry your team lost, Pete. Ref shoulda had Smith down by contact well before he stretched out that ball. Musta been watching the cheerleaders, not the game.

"Anyway, you put on a phenomenal display tonight and during the entire season. Fifteen tackles per game this season and stopping Smith twice tonight; at least two stops in my book. Impressive. Great work as a tight end, too. Your blocking is textbook. I wish our tight ends blocked as well. If you have some time, I'd like to talk with you some about coming to SC to play for the Trojans."

The week after the championship game college coaches, scouts, agents, well-wishers, and friends expressing sympathy over the loss filled the Stein's answering machine and Pete's cell phone inbox to capacity, not to mention inundating their email accounts. Even Julie's office phone was clogged with 42 messages the Monday after the game, while Sandy fielded 19 calls. Julie suspected that Sandy turned away some calls, having decided that taking messages from college coaches did not quite fall within her job description. Julie couldn't blame her. More than 40 colleges were interested in the middle linebacker who saved the Los Angeles City Championship for Santa Maria once—and almost twice.

"I think Pete could be a starter for us in a couple of years," the Arizona State defensive coach said. He phoned Julie one afternoon as she tried to read about plotting in Lajos Egri's *The Art of Dramatic Writing*. Plotting was one of her weaknesses.

"Best linebacker I've seen in years, bar none. Great athlete. Phenomenal combination of size, speed and athleticism."

"Athleticism?" Julie frowned at the unfamiliar term.

"Right."

Julie wondered if there was something called 'intelligentism' for aspiring doctors, lawyers and scientists, 'businessism' for aspiring moguls and 'religiousism' for aspiring rabbis and priests.

"Is he totally focused on becoming a pro football player?"

"He plays basketball and baseball, but football is his first love."

"In that case, I'd be right proud to see him come to Tempe to play for the Sun Devils."

"He's got another year of high school left," Julie warned, having only recently mastered the intricacies of high school football and finding herself adrift amidst the complexities and made-up language of college ball.

"That's fine. It'll give him time to put on a few pounds."

"He's 6' 2" and 195 pounds," she countered, wondering how big her little boy should be at 17 years of age.

"Another 25, say 30 pounds will put him right in the ballpark to be an impact player."

"Isn't he already an 'impact player'?" Julie abandoned trying to read her book and talk football-ese at the same time.

"Sure he is—at the high school level, but if he wants to play at the next level, in college, especially for a top program, he needs to top 200 as a linebacker and it better all be muscle and he better maintain his speed."

The other calls came from Oregon, Minnesota, Nevada, Florida, Michigan and Michigan State, Washington and Washington State,

Arkansas, Nebraska, and so many other schools Julie couldn't keep them straight. Pete had a list taped to his bedroom wall with checks for each time each school phoned, sent a card or letter, or emailed. As the checks proliferated, all the schools sounded the same to Julie, as if Pete was a product they all knew intimately, down to his shoe size—which they knew, too. They even used the same words and phrases. If one more coach told her Pete was a 'blue-chip prospect' she had decided to ask them what exactly the term meant.

"Jayden is already 11 pounds heavier than I am," Pete reported at breakfast through a mouthful of hot buttered toast. Pete had recovered rapidly from his devastation over the loss under the deluge of collegiate praise and attention.

"Aren't you faster?" Julie asked, skimming the application for a summer writer's workshop at the University of Iowa. It was the top creative writing program in the country, but she couldn't abandon Pete for two weeks. He could spend the time with his father, but Julie didn't want to surrender even two weeks of one of the last summers Pete would be at home to her ex-husband. Iowa would have to wait. "I thought you beat Jayden in the 40."

"By a second, but I could barely stop Smith. College backs are going to be bigger and stronger than Smith, especially the power backs. And in the pros....I was watching Adrian Peterson last weekend. He's a tank. I really need to bulk up. I have my off-season work cut out for me." He continued to shovel eggs, bacon, sausage, toast and a high-calorie, muscle-building shake Julie had approved into his mouth as if he hadn't seen food in a month.

"More eating and more working out?" Julie asked, as she nibbled on an English muffin with just a hint of butter. She envied Pete. She had never been told to gain weight in her life.

"Yeah, besides the winter and spring traveling teams, weekend camps and summer training camp." He made it sound like a dream schedule.

"What about basketball and baseball? And school?"

"I'll keep my grades up."

"Don't talk with your mouth full. When's your first camp this winter?"

He nodded to acknowledge her admonition, but chose to keep eating instead of answering. He had muscle to gain.

Other things may change us,
but we start and end with family.

—Anthony Brandt, US musician, b. 1961

Julie combed her shoulder-length wavy black hair to a glossy sheen. She checked her makeup in the rear-view mirror, applying an extra dab of lipstick, but not too much to her too-thin lips. Her mascara highlighted her black eyes well and she needed no rouge on her cheeks, since her skin appeared to have a permanent healthy tan, a gift from her Jewish ancestors. She grimaced at the few wrinkles around her eyes that had come with her forties, but a touch of foundation hid them as effectively as if they had never existed.

Stepping out of her neon-yellow VW Beetle into a warm December day, she straightened her simple black, knee-length skirt. With the white silk blouse, it had long been his favorite outfit on her. She held a stapled set of pages in her hand. Closing her eyes for a moment and letting out a deep breath to calm herself, she strode across the parking lot and into the three-story building in Cardiff-by-the-Sea, just up the coast from San Diego.

Pausing outside room 326, Julie knocked on the open door.

No answer.

She knocked again.

No answer.

She poked her head through the open doorway and stepped inside. The room faced south. The large single window had its blinds open, admitting a stream of warm, bright sunlight. Even with the window closed, Julie could smell the salt-tinged air from the ocean. The bed, positioned to allow anyone lying in it to see out the window with its view across the city to the Pacific, had been made, a quilt embroidered with a blue and white Mariner's star aligned on top.

A gleaming white door led to the bathroom while along one light-blue wall stood a pine bookcase overburdened with paperbacks, a 24-inch television on a pine stand, and a six-drawer pine bureau with three *Writer's Digest* magazines lying on top. Seated in a comfortable overstuffed chair next to a round table with a glass and chrome light on it, sat Ezra Stein.

"Hi, Dad," Julie called, beaming.

He looked up and said, "Hello"—no recognition in the word.

She fought back the depression she felt every time she came to see him. "I'm Julie, your daughter," she explained patiently, sitting on the edge of the bed.

No matter how often she visited, every time she came she had an image in her mind of her dad as he had been when she had been a little girl: his shoulders as wide as a door, his back straight, and his arms thick, darkened with black hair, matching the dense, unruly mass on his head. She knew he was now in his late seventies, yet every visit she was shocked by what she saw: a withered man with sparse white hair and a weathered, age-spotted face with pale yellow skin. His thoracic spine curved, giving him a stoop. Blue veins stood out on his hands, which were beginning to shows symptoms of arthritis. Strands of white stood out amidst the black hair on his arms.

"Julie, Julie," he repeated, searching for recognition. Maybe if Pete had come, her father would have recognized them together. Unfortunately, Pete had decided at the last minute to take his girlfriend Amanda rollerblading.

Julie saw a novel, Barry Unsworth's *Pascali's Island*, one of her father's favorites, open on his lap. Occasionally on a good day he could still read. Often she read to him one of her stories, as she had brought today, or a chapter from one of her novels. Occasionally he understood them.

"Julie," he said, recognition dawning. Something connected along the neural pathways amongst the senile plaques that had destroyed much of his cognitive ability and memory while distorting what remained. Looking over at her with an expectant child-like smile he asked, "How's your latest novel selling?"

Julie returned his smile, overjoyed at his recognition, but tinged with a soul-searing sorrow. "Well, Dad, very well. Thanks for asking."

Her father sighed and looked down. "That's something I always wanted to do; write a novel. Never had the time, though. With you kids, the business and all, never had the time." He looked back over at her. "I'm so proud of you, so very proud of my Julie, the novelist."

Julie forced herself to continue smiling. Her fingers crinkled the paper of the unpublished story in her hand as her grip tightened, whitening her knuckles.

He looked down at the novel in his lap and asked, frowning, "What's this thing?"

A musician must make music,
an artist must paint, a poet must write,
if he is to be ultimately at peace with himself.

—Abraham Maslow, US psychologist,
1908-1970

In her office at the Neurosurgical Institute, Julie wrote checks for her father's nursing home, Pete's college fund, her nieces' and nephews' college funds, and a large one for supplemental medical malpractice insurance. Only obstetrics rivaled neurosurgery for rapidly escalating insurance premiums. The hospital covered the premiums, which could top $1 million a year, but Julie paid for the supplemental plan, the premiums for which had shot up 50 percent in three years.

With her bank account well drained, she turned to analyze the data from her clinical trial for the treatment of Alzheimer's. The data looked promising, even though it was just a Phase I trial to test whether the drug combination was safe. Even so, it was hard not to be hopeful, even excited.

"Feel like lunch today?" Rick Severn asked.

Julie took in the pair of stately brunettes in tight blouses, thigh-length dresses and heels who waited just behind Severn at her doorway. They looked more like models than pharmaceutical reps.

"Thanks, but I have some data to go over," Julie replied with a knowing smile.

"Orsino's." Severn let the name roll off his tongue like the name of a vintage wine. "The finest food and drink." Slipping into her office, he leaned over her desk to whisper, "And free." His smile approached that of a five year old on the eve of his sixth birthday party.

"Tempting, but I think I'll pass."

"I pray my amygdala can handle the disappointment," Severn said with mock sincerity.

"If it can't, I'll transplant a new one for you."

"Can you do that?"

"I'd give it a try," Julie said and smiled up at Severn before adding, "in you."

Severn closed his eyes and clutching his chest moaned, "Harsh, so harsh."

"Did you get a chance to read that novel I loaned you?"

"*Lie in the Dark*? Not the greatest mystery, but the stuff about Sarajevo during the war was fascinating. Thanks."

"I have one by Somerset Maugham you might like, about a doctor, *Of Human Bondage*. Old, but powerful."

"Sounds like a possibility."

"I'll bring it in and leave it on your desk. Have fun at lunch."

"You know I will, my dear," Severn said, leaving to accompany his beguiling escorts to lunch.

Sandy, Julie's assistant, asked through the open doorway, "Why don't drug reps ever ask management assistants to lunch?"

"MAs don't decide which drugs to buy," Julie replied. "But I'll take you out for lunch the next time I don't have a long surgery or a lunch meeting."

"In late July then," Sandy said with a knowing smile. Then, serious, added, "Mrs. Croft's here again."

"Does she have an appointment?"

"No, but she's here all the same."

"Send her in," Julie said, with a resigned sigh.

"Good afternoon, Dr. Stein," Mrs. Croft said as she bustled in, struggling with a large bulky object wrapped in a worn patchwork quilt and held together with twine that teetered on a dented luggage cart. The twine dropped long strands of fiber on Julie's carpet every time Mrs. Croft moved.

"Good afternoon," Julie said, rising from behind her desk. "Is Mr. Croft alright?"

"Fine. Still painting night and day."

Mrs. Croft undid the twine and unwrapped the quilt, releasing from the bundle a dozen paintings of various sizes. Julie winced inwardly as she recalled her parting comment at their last meeting about the lack of art in the office.

"This is one of his earlier works," Mrs. Croft mentioned, leaning a 20" by 30" framed canvas against the wall. Blotches of blue, purple and red were applied here and there. Julie guessed it was supposed to be a lily pond, but she wouldn't have bet a cappuccino on it.

"Was Mr. Croft a professional artist?" Julie asked as Mrs. Croft arrayed the other paintings around the office against bookshelves, filing cabinets and beneath the long windows. Julie wondered how she was going to get out of this. Maybe she could buy one and slip it behind a filing cabinet before giving it as a present to someone she was obligated to, but despised.

"No, he wasn't a professional, not by a long shot. He just dabbled." Mrs. Croft placed the last painting under the x-ray light box.

Julie looked at the other paintings. Unlike the first painting, they were easily recognizable: amongst them a chestnut horse in a field; a heron diving into the ocean near a row of surfers awaiting the next wave; and a mountain meadow. They were rather well done. She glanced at the early painting and then at the others. There was a marked difference in style and, although Julie was far from being an art expert, a vast difference in their artistic merit. "Did he paint these since he's been in the clinical trial?"

"Yes. Since he's been on those drugs of yours he's been painting like a man possessed, as if he was actually getting paid for it."

Julie stood amazed before one of the paintings that Mrs. Croft had leaned against her filing cabinet. "They're good."

"I don't know about such silliness, but people say he's much better now than before he caught Alzheimer's."

"Did he paint after he was diagnosed but before he started taking the medications for the trial?"

"No. He couldn't remember what a paintbrush was for, let alone use one." Mrs. Croft stood back, eyeing her husband's work. "Well, can you help me out?"

Julie frowned, her mind on the effects of the trial's drug regimen on Alzheimer's disease. "I don't follow...."

"I mean, if you'd be so kind, can you take some of these off my hands? I can't be paying for paint and brushes and canvases and frames, and still put food on the table, let alone add to my tea cup collection."

Julie suppressed a smile and, scanning the offerings, several of which caught her eye, pointed at an Impressionistic painting of an astronomer by candlelight poring over manuscripts, and said, "I'll take that one."

After Mrs. Croft had bustled out with her artistic load, Julie told Sandy, "There's a painting in my office. Can you ask Facilities Management to come hang it beside the light box?"

"You're soft heart's going to get you into trouble," Sandy warned with a motherly smile.

"Already has; I am divorced," Julie said with a wry grin. "I'll be over in the lab at the PI meeting."

"If you have a sec," Sandy said, causing Julie to pause on her way to meet the other principal investigators. "The Budget Office called. They said they couldn't process our last batch of lab invoices."

"Why not?"

"You don't have a Form 2366: Capital Billing Authorization."

"First I've heard of it."

"They said you should have filled it out eight years ago when you joined Mount Hermon."

"I've been signing off on invoices for hundreds of thousands of dollars for eight years and they decide because I don't have a form in my file, I can't sign off on anything any more?"

"That's right," Sandy said, swiveling back and forth in her black chair, which wheezed asthmatically.

"Can you get the form?"

"I've got an email out to Reprographics, who are supposed to supply the forms."

"Great. Thanks." Julie turned to hurry away from the paperwork problem and toward the lab.

"If you've been embezzling from the lab, I'll keep quiet for a small cut."

"How small?" Julie called back over her shoulder.

"Just a measly five figures."

"Write up a check request, I'll sign it and you can try submitting it."

College football is a sport that bears
the same relation to education
that bullfighting does to agriculture.

—Elbert Hubbard, US editor, writer
and publisher, 1856-1915

Julie took a break from preparing latkes; the shredded potato, Matzo meal and onion pancakes fried in oil for Hanukkah. Although Pete was no longer a little boy, they still celebrated the Festival of Lights, at least to the extent of lighting a menorah and eating latkes drenched in applesauce. Pete loved latkes and Julie figured her diet and training regimen for the LA Marathon could allow for treats on religious holidays, which included devouring some See's chocolates a grateful ex-patient had sent her for Christmas.

As she entered Pete's room, Julie glanced over at the Bears number 54 jersey she had given Pete for Hanukkah. She had bought it at a charity auction for the South Los Angeles Free Clinic where she volunteered. Pete had given her a crushing hug when he had torn open the package and beheld the signed jersey from his hero, middle linebacker Brian Urlacher. Pete had debated whether to frame it or wear it; the later option barely won out in the end. Now he wore it most days. He had given her three novels, Richard Wright's *Native Son*, Graham Greene's *The Heart of the Matter* and Walker Percy's *The Moviegoer*, which moved her to within five books of completing her collection of The Modern Library's 100 Best Novels. She gave him a hug in return for his thoughtful gifts.

At his desk, Julie smiled in disbelief as she flipped through the University of Arkansas's red-accented book. Within a week after the championship game, brochures began to arrive for Pete with letters from defensive and head coaches from colleges across the country. Most were as thick as a historical novel and every page was four-color and glossy. In hyperbole-laden text and artistic images of receptions, tackles, touchdowns, stadiums, weight rooms, imposing stone and brick buildings, and well-built cheerleaders, each extolled the virtues, traditions, glorious past successes and predicted near-certain glowing futures of each school's football program.

She had never thought her son would ever play football but then again she had never planned to marry an ex-collegiate football player. "You'd think the football program was the entire university."

"Most people only know a college because of its team," Pete said, flipping through UCLA's booklet and stopping to admire with widening eyes the cheerleading squad of beaming girls with long hair, longer legs and toothy smiles that made Julie think they looked hungry. An appropriately diverse mix of every major ethnicity, Julie thought the cheerleaders were all prettier than she remembered anyone she knew in college ever being. Then again, UCLA was right next to Hollywood and who knew how much Photoshopping had gone into making each beauty look like the perfect co-ed.

"College is supposed to be about education and learning," Julie said.

"Yeah, learning to read an offense, tackle a back in the flats and blitz a quarterback who has good lateral movement," Pete said with a grin.

Julie dropped the Arkansas guide onto Pete's desk with a thunk. "Don't forget, you're going to college to get a degree."

"I wish they gave degrees in football."

"Pete, few college players ever make it to the pros."

Pete closed the UCLA brochure as he folded down the corner of the cheerleader page and said, "About 8 in 10,000 high school seniors who play football make it to the NFL. One in 50 college players are drafted and make it onto a pro team, or at least get the chance to try."

"How did you know that?"

"I looked it up a long time ago." Pete glanced up at his astounded mother. "I wanted to know the odds."

Julie smiled, but she knew that even if he knew the odds, Pete would believe that he would be one of the 8 in 10,000. "If you aren't one of the lucky few, what do you want to study in college?"

"Football."

"I mean something that will get you a job."

"Football."

"I mean a real job; something with a regular paycheck."

"Football."

"That's not a real job."

"It's the only thing I'm interested in," Pete said simply, as if it was a self-evident truth. He inspected the USC Song Girls displayed individually and in a group on a two-page spread of glossy images in Southern Cal's booklet.

"I know for a fact that football's not the only thing you're interested in."

Pete frowned.

"You're also interested in girls," Julie said, ruffling his short curly black hair with her hand.

Pete sighed and said, "Not many jobs in that field, either."

With the exception of women, there is
nothing on earth so agreeable or necessary to
the comfort of man as the dog.

—Edward Jesse, *Anecdote of Dogs*, 1880

January

In a navy blue tracksuit with three white stripes down the outside of each leg, Julie jogged down the sidewalk along Veterans Park near her house. The sun was only half an hour old, its rays still fresh and clean as they filtered through the jacarandas and eucalyptus trees, the Los Angeles smog yet to deaden their golden sheen. She rounded the corner of the park, glancing at a bed of flowers as the Eagles "Hotel California" played in her iPod earphones.

"Woo-oof!"

Julie dodged to the right, narrowly avoiding a battleship-grey terrier as she landed on the edge of the sidewalk. Stumbling, she came to a halt on the grass verge between the sidewalk and the street. A straight-backed man in his late thirties or early forties wearing a dark brown leather jacket, blue jeans and bright white sneakers held the leash of the startled canine.

"I'm extremely sorry," he was saying as Julie pulled off her earphones. "Mac was startled."

Rigid and alert, the muscular terrier eyed Julie warily.

"No harm done," she said, putting weight on her foot to test her ankle.

She looked up at the man. His dark eyes were as clear and alert as his terrier's. He had broad shoulders that filled out his unzipped jacket. His back was straight even as he leaned on a pale-wood cane that shone with layers of shellac.

"Is he a Scottie?" Julie asked, glancing down at the dog, which still eyed her with wary caution and undisguised suspicion.

"Yes, he is."

"I thought they were black."

"Usually. Come here, Macduff." The man hauled in the brindle dog and then scooped the purebred off its sturdy paws and into his arms. The dog looked far from happy with the turn of events. "A few, a very fine few Scotties are brindle, like Mac." The man held the dog out toward Julie.

She reached out her closed fist and let the dog imperiously sniff the back of her hand. Having been deemed worthy, the terrier lowered his head so she could scratch the regal cranium just behind the erect, tufted ears.

"Are you sure you're alright?" he asked.

"Fine, thanks." She had been more startled than hurt.

"We better let the nice lady continue her jog, Mac," the man told his canine companion as he set the dog down on the sidewalk.

Julie smiled as she began to put her earphones back on.

"I'm Alan McGhee."

"Julie Stein." She did not shake hands. His hands were full with leash and cane.

"A pleasure. Have a nice day, Julie Stein." He turned and, led by his distinctive terrier with the curved, erect tail, limped with his cane around the corner of the park and out of sight behind a sloping hill covered with annuals, bougainvillea and white-tufted pampas grass.

Julie watched him go, the way he had said her name still in her ears, as if the deep voice had filled each ear to its capacity, leaving behind a warm, welcoming feeling.

"Scans are complete," Hsu announced as he strolled into Julie's office at the Neurosurgical Institute lugging two thick, black binders.

"Great," Julie said, closing the short story she was writing on her computer and opening web access to the medical center's imaging files. The last thing she wanted was her research team to discover that she wrote fiction. If they found out, word would reach Baxter. She had no doubt he would view such scribbling as a sure sign she lacked dedication as a surgeon, researcher and clinician and, as he often told her only half in jest, an emerging leader in the field of Alzheimer's research. Sandy knew of Julie's literary pursuits, but a good management assistant knew never to talk about a boss's private business and Sandy was an extremely good management assistant.

"The MRIs show a reduction in plaques," Hsu reported.

Julie slid a pack of cigarettes—she had to quit...again—off her desk and into a drawer as she opened her trial patients' scans on her computer. Hsu came around her desk to view the scans. By comparing previous scans to the current ones on a split screen, she noted a decrease in the identity-destroying senile plaques in the cerebral cortex that were the major indicator of Alzheimer's.

Sandy darted in and deposited a stack of mail on the corner of Julie's desk. "You might want to look at this one," Sandy said, prodding an envelope off the top of the stack toward Julie.

Picking up the already opened envelope, Julie pulled out a piece of coated card-stock cradled in a folded piece of heavy bond paper. She frowned. "What is it?"

From the door on her way back to her cubicle, Sandy called, "A golf score card."

"Why's someone sending you a scorecard?" Hsu asked. "You taking up golf?"

Julie scanned the penciled numbers scrawled under each hole and, on the far right, the number 92 neatly circled. Beneath it, someone had printed the word, "Thanks" with a shaky hand, and then a name she could just make out. "It's from Tom Morris."

"Who's that?" Hsu asked, casually curious.

"A patient I operated on in November. I removed a pituitary tumor so he could see to play golf."

"Looks like it worked."

"It was cancerous, but I resected 99.9 percent of it. Chemo and radiation took care of the rest."

"Is 92 any good?"

"Ninety-nine point nine," Julie corrected Hsu.

"No, I mean is 92 a good golf score?"

Realizing that Hsu could care less about resection rates, Julie shrugged in answer to his question and opened the folded white paper. "He says his goal is to shoot his age. He used to be a 4 handicap—whatever that means—but he thinks shooting an 81 shouldn't be too hard, and every year it takes, it gets easier."

Julie slid the card and note back into the envelope and set it aside for safekeeping. She turned her attention back to the scans. "These look great."

"Looks even better on the Aurora system," Hsu reported as he stood looking over Julie's shoulder at her monitor. "You can see even more of the plaques receding."

"What about the other tests?"

"Not so good," Hsu admitted, coming back around her desk and sitting across from Julie with the thick binders on his lap. Everything in a clinical research trial had to be documented, usually in several places. Hsu flipped his long, black bangs out from in front of his eyes. "Seven subjects have bone density loss, five have elevated liver levels of AST and ALT, nine have hypertension, and most have reported headaches, dry metallic mouth, stomach upset, and minor ailments, including a few rather vivid hallucinations."

"Let me see." Hsu handed her the lab results. She saw nothing serious, but as she went through each case she jotted down drugs and treatments to prescribe to ensure that none of the conditions apparently caused by the clinical trial's drug cocktail became serious.

As a couple walked past her open office door, Julie glanced up to see Rick Severn saunter past with a pharma rep, his hand low on her back, dangerously close to her derriere. He carried a shopping bag in his other hand probably filled with a few small gifts from the drug company: pens, pads, mugs, and maybe even a pair of Lakers floor seats.

"Memory, both short- and long-term is improving in most of the subjects," Hsu said as he looked through the second thick binder on his lap.

Julie stopped and glanced at the painting by Mr. Croft, which now hung on her wall beside the light box. "How are they doing on the creativity tests?"

Hsu flipped some pages, flipped back to a tab and reported, "Very well. One even came up with a creative answer to the story about the locked, empty room in which the guy is found who'd hung himself, but with the noose too high for him to have reached it by himself."

"I liked the patient who said he stood on a block of ice and waited for it to melt. That's patience."

"That's nothing. A patient I had when I was at UBC suggested the dead man stood on a block of rotten wood full of termites and waited for the termites to eat all the wood so the guy could hang himself. That's real patience."

Julie laughed. "Do termites eat wood faster than ice melts?"

"I'll devise a study to investigate that question for you to submit to the NIH right away," Hsu said with mock seriousness. Julie liked working with Hsu. He was bright, attentive to detail and never let an opportunity to laugh pass.

"What was the latest creative answer?" Julie asked.

"The patient said the guy was in Australia, which is down-under, so the room was upside down with the noose laying on the floor. The guy put the noose around his neck and waited for the Earth to rotate to make the room right side up—the floor becoming the ceiling."

"Creative," Julie said, laughing, "But the Earth doesn't turn that way."

"We don't grade for realism, just the number of explanations."

*Sectional football games have the glory and
the despair of war, and when a Texas team
takes the field against a foreign state, it is an
army with banners.*

—John Steinbeck, US novelist and
Nobel Laureate, 1902-1968

"Hey, Tomlinson," Jayden Andrews yelled as he strode into the high school's weight room. Although football season was over, most of the players, at least any with collegiate aspirations, continued to train and workout throughout the winter, spring and summer. Other varsity athletes also used the room, but today Pete was alone, save for Manny Ortiz, a skinny sophomore safety who rode an exercise bike in the corner.

Pete finished his set of bench presses and sat up, wiping sweat off his face with a dark green Santa Maria High Spartans towel.

"You going to Jen's barbeque this afternoon?" Jayden asked Pete.

"Nah, going to workout again late this afternoon."

"Your own little two-a-days, huh?"

"Yeah."

"What about Amanda?"

"She's going, I think."

"Without you?"

"Yeah," Pete said, fighting against changing his mind.

"You must love football a helluva lot to miss a chance to spend a night with that body."

With a rueful smile, Pete asked, "You going?"

"Sure. Sharon and her sister are coming along. Should be fun," Jayden said with a leer. "Threesome here we come."

Pete rose and took a long swig of water.

"Got anything on the playoffs this weekend?" Jayden asked.

"A buck fifty on the Giants."

Jayden nodded, considering Pete's choice of teams. "Any letters of interest?" Jayden asked as he stretched his hamstrings by leaning against a wall beside a poster that proclaimed "Whatever It Takes!!!"

"A few," Pete said, striding over to an arm-curl machine. He glanced over at the sophomore Manny, who was listening, but trying not to look like it. "Mostly phone calls and brochures in the mail."

"I'm up to two dozen," Jayden said as he continued stretching the other major muscles and tendons in his 206-pound body. "Probably get 50 before the season starts."

"Letters?"

"Yeah."

"They promise anything?" Pete tried to sound only as casually interested as Jayden.

"They can't this early, but they basically say I can have a spot on their team if I have as good a senior year as I had last year. They're interested in me for basketball and baseball, too, but I want to play football." Jayden came over as Pete started his curls. "I'm sure you're getting the same sort of thing."

Pete fell silent. Although he and Jayden were teammates in football, basketball and baseball, Pete had never liked him. Pete did like Jayden to a certain degree, but it was a liking that went against his will. Jayden was too confident, too smooth and too in control. Pete had never seen Jayden take a penalty out of anger, let alone an unsportsmanlike call. Tall, muscular and with short-cropped blond hair, Jayden would have been right at home in a magazine story devoted to the perfect California teenager. He had a way about him that people liked. He was hard to dislike, but with a cheerleader girlfriend, wealthy parents, a new black BMW coupe, and a tight group of friends who worshipped him, a part of Pete just didn't like him.

"You're going to a top program, aren't you?" Jayden asked, starting to warm-up on a treadmill. For Jayden, such a course had been predestined since he was conceived. His father had gone to Nebraska during one of their heydays and become a star cornerback before playing a couple of years in the NFL. A knee injury ended his promising career.

"Sure." Pete tried to sound confident.

"No promises yet?"

"Not yet," Pete admitted with a challenging glance at the sophomore Manny. Pete finished a set of curls and swigged down more water.

"Damn," Jayden said, noticing Pete's water. "I forgot to take my vitamins." Jayden stepped off the treadmill and disappeared into the locker room. He returned and, popping two white, octagonal pills into his mouth, chugged down water from a white plastic bottle with "Huskers" emblazoned in red across it.

Jayden resumed his treadmill run while Pete continued his strength training and Manny rode on, sweat staining his grey Spartans T-shirt. The clink and squeak of the machines and the three boys' puffs now and then were the only sounds in the weight room. Their sweat began to tinge the air with a pungent aroma.

"They say I need to put on 15 or 20 pounds," Pete spat out, as if it left a bad taste in his mouth.

Manny said, "I need to gain at least 40." He fell silent as Pete and Jayden cast stern looks in his direction. Sophomores never spoke unless spoken to.

"You can do that," Jayden told Pete, as if it was nothing. "They say I could add a few pounds in the next year—maybe five or so; no problem at all."

Pete wished he was as confident. He worked out and worked out and worked out—and the pounds never came. Already all muscle, Jayden had grown over the past couple of years from a lanky kid into a broad-shouldered giant.

"Coach mentioned there's a new linebacker, Joe Cain, transferring in next fall from some school in Texas; All State," Pete said, making sure there was little concern, let alone any trace of worry in his voice.

"Only thing they grow in Texas are steers and loudmouths," Jayden said. "Remember that linebacker, Bosworth, way back in the seventies?"

"Eighties."

"Whatever. All mouth. Out of the pros in a couple of years. Now he's an actor or something in straight-to-DVD movies."

"He played for Oklahoma, not Texas."

"Same thing, east of here; hot, flat, flyover land. Don't worry, Tomlinson. You and I are the linebackers on this team. That's certain."

"Who's worried?"

Julie stood just outside a door that led to the hall across from the Ronald Reagan UCLA Medical Center's main auditorium. She sucked on a cigarette: her last. She had to quit, even if she was down to only a couple—or four—or five—a day. Smoking was bad for her and a bad example for Pete. She was supposed to be training for the LA Marathon. On top of that, a doctor should be the last person to smoke. She shook her head at her lack of willpower against nicotine. Why had she ever started smoking?

"They're ready for you," Sandy said, opening the door and looking out at her boss. "I thought you'd quit."

"Which time?"

Julie followed Sandy back into the auditorium. She hoped her make-up was holding up, that her white blouse, black jacket and slacks were spotless, and that her hair had maintained its position the last time—the tenth—she'd fixed it in the bathroom mirror just before she and Sandy had found the auditorium.

More than 100 physicians and researchers in white lab coats, dark blue or green scrubs and a sprinkling of suits sat in various states of repose on gray plastic chairs in the high-ceilinged lecture hall. Save for four women, the audience was male. A large screen behind the podium displayed a PowerPoint slide: University of California, Los Angeles, Department of Neurosurgery Grand Rounds, "Promising Advances in Alzheimer's Treatment," Julie Stein, MD, PhD, Mount Hermon Medical Center, Los Angeles, CA.

"A world-renowned expert on the treatment of Alzheimer's and other neural degenerative diseases, Dr. Stein is a great hope to millions suffering from Alzheimer's," Gordon Jakes, the Chair of Neurosurgery at UCLA said from a podium at the front of the hall. "I've known her for more than 15 years and there is no one better in which to place the hope of millions of Alzheimer patients." He glanced over at Julie as she waited near a side door and fought the temptation to chew a fingernail. "She has always impressed me, except for her decision to accept a position at Mount Hermon and not here at UCLA."

The audience chuckled.

"Rhodes Scholar, researcher with articles in every journal worth mentioning, including five, yes five in *The New England Journal of Medicine*, surgeon with the finest pair of hands I've ever seen, teacher, marathoner, and someone who spends her vacations doing surgery for Doctors Without Borders and Operation Smile in places even Marines avoid, as well as volunteering her expertise at the South Los Angeles Free Clinic, it is my pleasure to introduce Dr. Julie Stein."

Julie shook Jakes' hand as she reached the lectern and surveyed the audience. "Thank you, Gordon. That was the kind of introduction my father would have liked and my mother would have believed."

Laughter. Good, she thought.

"I'm here to share with you some preliminary data on my research team's study into treating Alzheimer's disease with a combination of drugs that influence the presenilin 1 and 2 genes in combination with controlling the calcium levels in brain cells," Julie said as she rested her left hand on the laptop atop the lectern to start the PowerPoint portion of her talk. "I hope you'll agree that we've had some excellent—albeit early—results from our Phase I trial, especially in the areas of memory, cognition and, most importantly since success in the area has been so elusive, in the area of creativity."

Take a breath, Julie told herself. Not so fast. She hated this. She had done it a hundred times, yet she still hated it. It reminded her of when she had first become a surgeon and discovered that she had to build a practice. Patients did not just come to you, no matter how well you did in medical school. Like every new surgeon, she had to go out to meet neurologists, internists, oncologists and other potential referrers, presenting talks, attending dinners and making a good impression on those who could send her patients. It had been hard, and something she had never realized a physician had to do. She learned how to do it, but never learned how to like it.

Facing the audience in the auditorium, she forced herself to slow down. "As you probably know, Alzheimer's disease has been identified as a protein misfolding disease due to the accumulation of abnormally folded A-beta and tau proteins in the brains of AD patients. The plaques are made of a peptide, called beta-amyloid, a protein fragment snipped from a larger protein called amyloid precursor protein or APP, which is believed to help neurons grow and repair themselves. In Alzheimer's disease, something causes APP to divide into fragments. One type of these fragments are beta-amyloids, which clump together to form the dense formations known as senile plaques. Therefore, our research focuses on protecting APP from damage, as well as dispersing or destroying the beta-amyloid clumps before they damage the brain. If we can protect the APP, we may save the brain from deterioration in the areas of cognition and creativity."

In his Brian Urlacher Bears jersey, Pete rushed into his bedroom after his workout, clicked on a Three Doors Down CD on his iPod stereo and powered up his red laptop on the bed. He typed in 'Joe Cain, linebacker/tight end, Texas' and waited an instant for the Internet search results. He took a swig of a protein shake he had grabbed from the fridge and clicked on a link that looked promising.

He skimmed a news story from *The Dallas Morning News* that extolled Cain's successes on the gridiron, as well as on the basketball court, baseball diamond and track. Pete found what he was looking for: Joe Cain, 6 foot 3. Pete was 6 foot 2, but an inch didn't matter much. Strength, reaction time and speed were keys to a great linebacker. Cain was 220 pounds. Pete's mouth fell open. He peered at the screen to make sure he had read what he thought he had read. He had: 220. Pete was 195.

Steeling himself for any more bad news, Pete read on. Cain was from Heatherdale High, which had won four Texas state championships, and was a division AAAAA school; the biggest and toughest division.

There had to be something to give Pete hope. He read on; Cain was a junior, same as Pete. With that extra 25 pounds, he had to be slower than Pete, at least Pete desperately hoped so. Pete read the rest of the article, but there was nothing beyond praise for Cain's athleticism, speed and dexterity. Hype, where were the stats?

Pete checked another story, then another, and finally found what he was looking for in *Texas Football* magazine, apparently the bible of Texas football: Cain was 4.55 for 40 yards. Pete was 4.8.

"Ugh," Pete moaned and threw himself back on the bed. He wasn't going to make the team next year; Cain would replace him.

You will never understand bureaucracies until you understand that for bureaucrats procedure is everything and outcomes are nothing.

—Thomas Sowell, US writer and economist, b. 1930

As they drove together back to Mount Hermon from UCLA, Julie resisted the temptation to smoke in Sandy's presence, even if they were in Julie's Beetle.

"I spoke with Reprographics," Sandy said.

Julie frowned as she changed lanes to get around an SUV turning down posh Rodeo Drive from Santa Monica Boulevard.

"They don't have the form anymore."

"What form?" Julie had been thinking about how to revise a short story that had just been rejected. She had to present the hero's central problem far earlier and make it more vital to him.

"Form 2366: Capital Billing Authorization."

Julie's frown deepened as she stopped for a red light. She could have caught the yellow, but she had already been forced to ask Sandy sweetly twice in the past year to complete online traffic school for her. It had only required a lunch at Orsini's each time in compensation; well worth the investment to avoid the time wasted to take the class.

"The form to allow you to sign off on lab expenditures of greater than $500," Sandy explained. She had been Julie's guide through the Mount Hermon bureaucracy since Julie's first day at the medical center.

"I've been signing off on lab expenditures of greater than $500 for eight years."

"Against Mount Hermon policy apparently."

"Reprographics doesn't have the form?" The instant the light turned green, Julie accelerated across the intersection.

"They stopped using it five years ago."

"Did you tell the Budget Office we can't get the form?"

"They said you can't sign off on any more expenditures until the form is signed by various bigwigs and is in your personnel file."

"So I don't have to sign invoices anymore? Great. That'll free up some time." Julie veered right onto Burton Way, with its broad, grassy meridian sporting magnificent jacarandas, palms and magnolias dating back to Beverly Hill's incorporation in 1906. "That should give me enough time to find a cure for Alzheimer's, master the intricacies of college football, and write the Great American novel, with time left over to win a Nobel Peace Prize or three."

"I spoke with someone in the Budget Office. She'll fax over someone else's Form 2366."

"That's nice," Julie said, not following Sandy's line of thought.

"We'll white out their information and put in yours."

"You're frighteningly devious. I'll have to try to get you a President's Award for that one."

"I'm still expecting my cut of the lab money you've been embezzling."

"It'll have to be a cash payment with unmarked bills made on a dark, stormy night in the parking structure," Julie said with a laugh. "Harder to trace that way."

"Any way I get it is fine."

Julie changed lanes and said, "I just bought a stack of new books you might like." Julie gestured back at the jumble of novels, how-to-write books, medical journals and bags sporting logos from a range of medical conferences covering the back seat and spilling onto the floor.

Sandy said, "I'll look through them when we get to the hospital."

"Borrow any you like."

"Severn's asking about a dinner this Saturday night," Sandy said, reading off her palm pilot.

"With who?" Severn always aroused her suspicions.

"A company offering a new drug to treat vasospasm."

"Pass."

"You could take a free meal once in a while. What would it hurt?"

"My integrity."

"Passed," Sandy said as she typed a reply on the pilot's tiny keyboard.

Julie's cell played the first few notes of U2's "I Still Haven't Found What I'm Looking For." It was Hsu, her researcher. She put in her earpiece as she turned up Doheny toward the medical center.

"One of the study's patients is in the ED," Hsu said.

"What happened?" Julie asked.

"Fell and broke his hip."

"Condition?"

"Should be fine."

"Not unexpected given the age of our patient population."

"No," Hsu replied, drawing out the word.

"It's not related to the trial, is it?"

"The x-ray showed advanced osteoporosis."

"Again, not uncommon in our patient population," Julie said, swinging around to pass a Honda hybrid that was turning right and was waiting for a pedestrian to cross the side street in front of it.

"It is uncommon when an osteoporosis test he had a year ago, before he started the study, showed no sign of it."

"I'll see him and then I'll meet you in the lab." As she pulled into one of the Mount Hermon parking structures, she asked Sandy, "Can you get me a cigarette out of my purse? I need one." She met Sandy's disapproving glare with steely resolve.

"Let's check every subject in the study for osteoporosis," Julie told Hsu as they sat in her tiny satellite office in the lab. She could hear techs working just outside her open door; pipettes clicking off test tubes, a magnetic stirrer whirring and someone washing beakers in a sink. A whiff of cleaning alcohol reached her nose.

Hsu said, "Some of the patients also have elevated blood pressure, elevated liver enzyme levels, and have reported headaches, diarrhea and dry mouth." He pushed his long, straight black hair out from in front of his black eyes. With his faded, frayed blue jeans, a U-2 *Rattle and Hum* T-shirt, a silver ear stud and necklace, and a face that made him look about twenty-five, Hsu didn't look like a forty-something principle investigator with a wife and two adorable, precocious kids. On top of that, Julie often found it hard to believe that Hsu had missed most of elementary school during the Cultural Revolution when schools in China had been shuttered. Even with a major gap in his formal education, he had come to America to earn a doctorate at Princeton before doing post-doctoral research at Cambridge University and securing a research position at the University of British Columbia. Julie heard about him and lured him away eight years ago to help lead her research group as a principal investigator.

"All the side effects sound manageable," Julie said, hoping nothing worsened.

"Couple of patients report some vivid hallucinations; roads going the wrong way, dogs changing color and a spouse who turned out to be someone else."

"I'm afraid to ask."

"Hopefully it wasn't during an intimate moment."

"Didn't you ask?"

"I do have some discretion," Hsu said haughtily, taking mock offense.

"You didn't about spreading that story about the experimental IUD."

"When the string for the IUD got caught in the woman's partner's foreskin and they had to call 9-1-1?"

"I wonder how they answered the door when they were still, well, attached."

"I was passing along important medical research information," Hsu said, failing to suppress his laughter.

"I doubt we'll be researching any IUDs in neurosurgery," Julie countered, but also started laughing. Settling down, she said, "I'll ask Bill Rogers over in psych about the hallucinations. He's done a pile of research on visual hallucinations."

"Couple of patients report auditory and olfactory hallucinations, too."

"Rogers will know who to consult about them. To be safe, let's check every subject's blood pressure, do an MRI of every subject to check for any changes in the brain, and bring in Jeff Conston to give them a thorough GI checkup. Charlie Woo can check their livers. I don't want any SAEs." A significant adverse event not only meant someone died, it also meant an in-depth review, which put a study at grave risk of being terminated.

As Mr. Sanderson lectured on how animals convert food into energy, Pete was focused on Sharon Fraser's tits. Her magnificent breasts filled out her bright yellow sweater like a pair of beacons to every breathing male in sight.

Sharon glanced at him and, realizing he was about to cross the border from open admiration to stalking-like stare, Pete turned his attention to the other side of the room. Maria Martinez was looking stunning today, her long copper legs revealed in all their shapely glory by a miniskirt of some soft, supple material that draped over her thighs most provocatively.

Pete had only taken Biology 11 because of his mom. When it had come time to select courses for his junior year, the school required him to take one science course. He had always done better in English, History and Government. He had little interest in any of the sciences, but his mom's enthusiasm for biology had tipped the scales so that at the last second as he filled out his course choices he checked biology. He had harbored a hope that biology would include some sex, but thus far there had been next to nothing about procreation, let alone sex. Now he realized that it had been a wise choice even without any sex since, interested or not, over the years he had soaked up a lot of useless facts about biology from his mom. He had earned an A on his midterm and that was after paying little, if any attention in class—at least little attention to the lectures. Sharon and Maria were another matter.

When Maria glanced at him and smiled, he returned the smile and then, thinking of his girlfriend, Amanda, shifted his attention to his training schedule in his notebook. He tried to see if he was neglecting anything. He had exercises and weight training for every major muscle group and many of the smaller ones if they were related in any way to football. He also blocked out time slots for cardio work and even some mental exercises he had found on-line to help him visualize plays and tackles he might have to make during a game.

"Pete, what is the cycle that allows living cells to turn oxygen into usable energy?" Mr. Sanderson's voice broke into Pete's training thoughts.

"The Kreb's cycle," Pete replied, thankful he had heard his name; more thankful still that he had known the answer.

The break in his thinking changed the course of his thoughts from training to Joe Cain. If Pete didn't shine during the August tryouts, Cain would replace Pete at one of the linebacker slots. Pete was certain he would be the one replaced and not Jayden, since Jayden was bigger, stronger and, Pete had to admit, better than Pete. If Pete noticed the slight difference, then he was certain the coaches would notice a monumental difference between them. The conclusion, Pete knew, was obvious: he had to beat Cain for the other spot.

Pete was already weight training and eating well to close the 25-pound difference between himself and Cain. He was running wind sprints to close the quarter-second difference between them in the 40. The more he thought about it, the more Pete knew that just running more and gaining more muscle wasn't going to shave time off his 40. In fact, although stretching was an integral part of his training regimen, there was the danger of becoming muscle-bound and slower as he gained weight, even if it was all muscle. There had to be a better way to sprint faster than by adding muscle. Ignoring the lecture, Pete sat on his lab stool and wrestled with the dire problem.

*Prey drive: the instinctive behavior of a
carnivore to pursue and capture prey.*

—S. Donald Mac, *Biology*, 45th Ed., 2012

February

Julie was jogging along the sidewalk lost in U2's *The Joshua Tree*, when a writhing gray mass slammed her sideways into the wet, clammy grass. Teeth sank into her left sneaker. Canines pierced her skin. She kicked. She scurried away on her backside to escape the ferocious pit bull. It did no good. The dog still had her foot secure in its mouth.

Terrified, she heard above the dog's snarls a higher pitched, fierce growl. Glancing to the left she saw her neighbor Alan McGhee hobbling toward her with his Scottish terrier in the lead.

Alan tied his snarling terrier's leather leash around a lamp standard and lunged toward the pit bull. He grabbed a hind leg and lifted. Even with its hind legs off the pavement, the pit bull would not release Julie's shoe. She could feel the teeth tear the skin off her foot as the dog clamped down harder to hold on. Pain coursed through her foot. Fear and panic welled up within her. Her body was covered in fear-induced sweat. She fought to wrench her foot out of the dog's mouth. She may as well have tried to pull her leg out of its socket. The dog twisted and shook with her foot in his mouth. Julie wiggled and scuttled along the ground. She fought to keep her leg at an angle that would avoid tearing any tendons or breaking any bones

Just as she feared the dog would succeed in ripping her foot off, Alan reached around with his free hand and slugged the dog in the nose. It had no apparent effect, save that the dog snorted. Alan punched again. The pit bull released its grip on Julie's shoe. The dog spun around with incredible speed to snarl, teeth barred and mouth spraying spittle, at Alan. Julie scrambled back out of the way on her hands and knees. Alan clung to the dog's hind leg.

"Call 9-1-1!" Alan yelled, twisting and turning to keep the pit bull from sinking its teeth into any part of him.

She called. Moving away from the battle, she quickly reported the situation. The calm operator said help was on the way. Julie yelled to Alan, "What should I do?"

"Secure Mac."

Julie came around behind the rearing, barking Scottie. She held the leash where it was tied to the lamp standard. Luckily, the terrier's ferocious snarling and lunging had only succeeded in tightening the knot.

The pit bull was still snarling, snapping and spinning, but was tiring. Alan held on, shifting to the left, then the right, forward and back to retain his hold on the dog's hind leg and to keep away from the dog's flashing white teeth. Spittle flew from the dog's mouth, its face contorted with rage.

Julie heard a siren over the raucous cacophony of the dogs. The electronic noise rose above the hurly burly of the canine battle. A police car came to a rocking stop at the curb. An officer bolted from the car.

"You alright, Miss?" the tall, gray-haired officer asked Julie.

"I'll be fine. Help him!" Julie yelled, gesturing at Alan as he struggled to hang onto the pit bull.

Before the officer could react, an orange animal control truck arrived. A portly Latino man in a tan shirt and dark green slacks slid out and sauntered over with a metal snare in his right hand. An aroma of institutional soap engulfed him. As he came, he surveyed the situation. He seemed far from surprised, let alone concerned by the situation. The animal control officer waited for his opportunity. Then in one fluid motion the officer ensnared the pit bull by its thick neck and, bending his knees to take the weight, lifted the writhing, thrashing, twisting dog into one of the white-doored holding kennels on the back of his truck. With long-practiced ease, the officer released the noose and withdrew the pole in one smooth motion as he double latched the door.

Julie hobbled over to thank her rescuer. "Are you alright?" she asked Alan above the continued barking of the pit bull in the truck and the Scottie secured to the lamp standard.

"Fine," Alan said, wincing. He sat on tiled steps leading up to a Craftsman house. Holding his knee, he grimaced. "How's your foot?"

Julie sat beside him on the step and, peeling off her torn runner and perforated, blood-stained sock, inspected two bloody gashes in her foot. "Alright. Thanks to you, I still have both feet." Looking at him as he held his knee, she asked, "What's wrong with your knee?"

"Twisted. That's my cane," he called to the police officer, as the patrolman picked up the cane, which had ended up in the gutter.

"Settle down Mac," Alan called to his agitated terrier. "It's alright now."

The Scottie was still barking excitedly in a heated argument with the pit bull, who continued to bark ferociously in reply from the truck. Alan accepted his cane from the officer and hobbled over to untie his dog's leash, which took some doing after Mac had pulled on it with such force. Reunited with his master, the Scottie jumped up and down, roaring with happiness and relief. The pit bull, deprived of another dog with whom to argue, quieted down.

"I don't know how I can thank you enough," Julie told Alan. "I hope your knee's alright. Sit down and let me check it."

Alan hesitated, but did what he was told. Julie felt, kneaded and manipulated his knee. Alan grimaced a couple of times, but after a few moments, Julie announced, "Apply ice 10 minutes every hour, ibuprofen to reduce the swelling, and you should be good as new in a few days."

"You should have someone take a look at that foot," he said, eyeing her bloody foot.

"I'll call an ambulance," the patrolman said, starting to reach for a mike clipped to the left breast of his dark-blue shirt.

"No, wait," she said. "I'll be fine."

The officer and Alan looked doubtful. Her foot had jagged gashes just below the toes, which dripped blood.

"I've had a tetanus shot within the past 10 years and these aren't large enough to require stitches. I can clean them at home and bandage them."

The officer and Alan still looked unconvinced.

"The last thing a hospital needs is another case in their ER. I can take care of it myself, I promise."

Still unconvinced, the officer's hand was still on his radio mike.

"I'm a doctor, alright? I'll take care of it." She smiled her sweetest smile, and Alan, who looked surprised, and the officer nodded.

The report for the police and animal control took a quarter hour. As they were finishing, a second squad car arrived with a slender, frail woman with silver hair in the passenger seat. She rushed over to the animal control truck to call reassurance to the pit bull in its kennel as the newly arrived police officer strode over to his colleague.

"Found her searching along Windsor for her dog," the second officer, a young, curly-haired Latino, reported. "She broke down when I said her dog attacked somebody."

"I'm so sorry, so terribly sorry," the woman said, her face a mask of anguish as she approached Julie and Alan. She walked with an uneven, staggering gait. Julie diagnosed a hip or neurological condition. "I was out walking Peaches."

"Peaches?" Alan interrupted in disbelief.

"The first day I had her as a puppy, she got into a bowl of peaches and ate every single one," the lady explained with a sweet smile of remembrance. The smile turned to a look of horror when she saw Julie's bloody foot. "Oh, my God, are you hurt?"

"Just minor puncture wounds," Julie reassured the woman. "Has she attacked people before?"

"No, no, no, absolutely not," the lady said, holding up a wrinkled, boney hand in dismay. "Peaches is all sweetness, belly rubs and tongue licks. She adores my grandchildren. I would never, ever keep a dog that was aggressive in any way."

"Then what happened?" Alan asked.

"I was talking to a neighbor, a squirrel ran past and Peaches backed out of her collar." Her words rushed out in an emotional torrent. "She was gone before I knew it. I've been frantic to find her for the past half hour; the longest half hour of my entire life."

"She probably saw you running past and thought you were prey," the first police officer told Julie. "Happens from time to time, especially with kids on bikes."

The lady swallowed, glanced over at the animal control truck in which her precious Peaches was imprisoned and asked, hand at her wrinkled throat, "I hope you aren't going to make them destroy my Peaches." Her eyes narrowed and her lips pursed as she fought back tears. After a snuffle, she said, "This was just a terrible, awful thing, but it'll never happen again, I swear. I'll get a harness for her and make sure she never slips her collar again. This has never happened before and, if it had, I'd have bought a harness long ago. I'd never want to lose my Peaches and she'd never hurt anyone. I'm so sorry, it's just that, well, Peaches is the only one I have now that Walter's gone."

Alan helped Julie toward her house, even as he hobbled along on his injured knee with his cane. Mac, tail erect, carriage challenging, strained against his leash. He looked as if he had just bested a pack of pit bulls singlehandedly.

"What did animal control say?" Julie asked.

"He said he'd check if there were any other reports on that dog," Alan said. "If not, unless we take the owner to court, she can get her dog back."

"You going to court?"

"You were the one attacked."

"You were the one who hurt your knee."

Alan considered. "I think she'll keep Peaches under control in the future."

Julie nodded and looked at Alan.

"What?" Alan asked, noticing her stare.

"Nothing." She kept staring.

"What?"

"Oh, you're just a softie, that's all."

Alan snorted. "Don't ever tell my men that; I'll be toast."

Alan helped her up the steps into her house and into her living room. Looking around at the seven six-foot bookcases that covered three of the room's walls, he asked, "You run a library?"

"I like to read."

Alan helped her to the sofa and found gauze, bandages and antiseptic to bandage her foot, all while she protested that he, with the sprained knee, should be the one resting.

"Anything else? Want the TV on?" Alan asked, glancing over at the flat screen mounted above the fireplace.

"There's nothing ever on I can stand, except *Booknotes, Nova* or *Frontline*. Could you get me the novel off my bedside table? Second door on the left down the hall."

He returned with Yann Martel's *Life of Pi*. He was reading the blurb on the back as he walked. "Sounds bizarre," he said as he handed her the paperback.

"A little, but it's a great story; very engaging."

"I'll have to read it some time."

"You can borrow it as soon as I'm finished it."

"I guess I better be going."

"Let's not meet like this again, if that's okay with you?" Julie said. She sat on the sofa, her foot bandaged and with a blue ice pack wrapped around it to reduce swelling. "A simple hello will suffice next time. The dogfight was completely unnecessary. If this escalation continues from a Scottie startling me when we first met, to a pit bull attacking me as a prelude to our second meeting, I shudder to think what will happen when we meet for a third time; a mauling by a Bengal tiger?"

"Not many Bengal tigers in Los Angeles."

"It just takes one."

"Take care of that foot, and I hope to see you out jogging again soon, sans pit bull or tiger."

"I hope your knee gets better soon."

"Probably set my recovery back some, but no worries."

"Recovery?"

Alan glanced at the cultured-stone fireplace. "I messed up my knee a while back."

When he added nothing more, she said, "I hope it heals soon."

"You want to train with me?" Adina Gebreyohannes asked Pete as he stood before her on the high school's black, cinder track one cool morning before school.

"You're the fastest one on the track team, right?" Pete asked, feeling awkward and nervous in his treasured Bears jersey and black shorts.

"For sprints, not distance," she said, her tall, slender body displayed in a singlet that proclaimed her All State in Track and Field. Sunlight glinted off the sheen of sweat on her forehead.

"Sprint's what I need."

"For what? Basketball? Baseball?"

"Football."

"I thought football was all about hitting people."

"Your time in the 40-yard dash is the single most important test used by college football coaches to evaluate players. It combines strength, speed, power, balance, coordination, and aerobic and anaerobic conditioning."

Adina raised an eyebrow and smirked.

Pete broke into a grin. "I've been reading up on how colleges recruit football players." He looked down for an instant, then looked up at her, meeting her dark eyes with a look that threw down a challenge to smirk at what he was about to say. "I want to play in college and then in the NFL."

"I don't know why anyone would want to play such a brutal game."

"I love it."

"The track team has to go to the Friday pep rally. It's boring."

Pete chuckled. He thought best not to mention that he spent most of the time at the rally eyeing the cheerleaders, the Lady Spartans. "I just love playing football."

"You'd never catch me even going to a game."

"Nothing keeps me from playing. I finished a game with a broken finger when I was a junior."

"That's crazy," Adina said, her face contorted with disgust.

"That's what my mom said," Pete said with a grin. "My dad, who played some college ball, understood."

"I just don't see the point."

Pete considered. "I just love it, every bit of it. I love making a perfect tackle or cutting through a gap between two linemen to sack the QB. I even like the coaches yelling at us at halftime if we're behind and if we're winning—nothing like it. I'm on a high for days."

Adina nodded thoughtfully. She stretched one of her legs by pulling her foot up behind her to her tight, red shorts and holding it while she stood on the other leg. Perfectly still, her straight, tensed leg looked like a dark marble column sculpted by a Renaissance master. "I still don't see why you want to train with me," she said releasing her foot and doing the same thing with her other foot. The other leg, Pete noticed, was just as muscled and sculpted as the first.

"I need to increase my 40 speed and I read that training with the track team can make you faster."

"Why don't you just talk to Coach and train with the team?"

"He said to work with you."

Adina frowned. "Why me?"

"You're a sprinter and getting off the blocks fast is the key in a sprint; same as going from a standing start to full speed is the key in football."

"There are other sprinters on the team."

"He said you're the fastest sprinter, hardest worker and you know the fundamentals better than anyone, and…."

"And?" she prompted with an elfish glint in her dark eyes.

Pete hesitated, but she kept waiting for an answer. "He said if I can keep up with you, I deserve to be in the NFL."

Adina nodded as she considered this series of compliments, jangling the bright rainbow of beads woven into her hair. She said, "I work hard."

"So do I."

"I like to train alone."

"He said that, too."

"Why would I want to train with you?"

Pete looked across the empty field as the morning sun peeked over the line of Italian cypresses on the edge of campus and, looking back at her, said with his best smile, "Company?"

*It is not a case we are treating;
it is a living, palpitating, alas, too often
suffering fellow creature.*

—John Brown, Scottish physician, 1735-1788

"One of your research subjects presented with a stroke," the ER doctor reported to Julie over the phone.

"Who?" Julie asked as she rolled over in her Queen-sized bed and peered through slit eyes at the clock on her bedside table: 2:35 a.m. Long a doctor, she had perfected the art of sounding awake when she was not.

"Danny Molina."

"Presentation?" She sat on the edge of the bed, her head resting on her hand to steady it as she blinked sleep out of her eyes. The wood floor was cold on her bare feet, even the one wrapped in a bandage from the dog bites, but the cold helped wake her up.

"Sudden-onset headache, slurred speech and blurred vision."

"Stroke."

"CT ruled out a hemorrhagic, but the MRI showed a clot in the left frontal lobe. Blood sugar level is normal. He's on oxygen and an IV."

"Thrombolysis?"

"Contraindicated: had surgery for a goiter in his neck three months ago."

"Who's on call?"

"Boardman. He wants to use the MERCI system to remove the clot, but wanted to check with you first in case your clinical trial might affect the decision to use it. He's prepping for surgery, so he asked me to call."

Julie tried to recall the success rate for the Mechanical Embolis Removal in Cerebral Ischemia Trial. The FDA had just approved the minimally invasive, mechanical method of removing clots, but Julie liked to do a little more research on new devices and drugs than just rely on the FDA. She was suspicious of any regulatory organization that was funded by the companies being regulated, let alone one where the staff left the organization to find lucrative jobs with the same companies they had been charged with regulating.

She ran through the drugs in her clinical trial, recalling drugs, treatments and procedures for which they were contraindicated. "I don't think the MERCI system is contraindicated for any of the trial drugs, but I'm far from certain. The drug combination hasn't been thoroughly tested. When's Boardman going in?"

"Patient is being prepped as we speak."

"Tell him it's okay by me, but I want to be there."

"First incision in 45 minutes."

"I'll be there in 30."

Twenty-six minutes later Julie limped out of the elevator toward the OR suites on the eighth floor of the medical center's north tower. In clogs to better accommodate her punctured foot and dark blue scrubs, she was ready to assist in the OR, if needed or at least to observe. As she reached out to push open the door to the hall that led to the operating rooms, Patrick Boardman, in scrubs and smelling of disinfecting soap, opened it from within.

"Ready?" she asked.

"He stroked out while we were wheeling him into the OR," the neurosurgeon said as he untied a surgical mask that hung around his pale neck.

Julie stopped. She felt the sense of futility and loss that still shot through her whenever she lost a patient, no matter how much she had trained herself over the years to compartmentalize her emotions in order to be able to do her job. Her ex-husband had often told her she showed about as much emotion as a rock, but showing emotions and feeling emotions were worlds apart.

Pushing the powerful feelings of futility and loss into a back corner of her brain, she felt them replaced by anger and frustration. Of all her patients to die of a stroke, why did it have to be one of the subjects in her clinical trial? Why, why, why? The subjects had been doing so well, their Alzheimer's symptoms receding rapidly.

She thanked Boardman for contacting her and turned to head for the elevators to get outside where she could smoke. As she limped down the hall, the thought crossed her mind unbidden that the LA Marathon was fast approaching. She was supposed to be training for it, assuming her foot healed in time. But, she thought, if you can't have a cigarette when you lose a patient, when can you have one?

Pete opened a door on the first floor of the tallest building west of the Mississippi, the U.S. Bank Tower, and stepped into the cool, dim stairwell. Manny Ortiz, the skinny, sophomore safety crowded in behind him.

"It's sure great that you asked me to train with you," Manny said, his words tumbling over each other in his enthusiasm.

"Just today," Pete cautioned, already regretting his impulsive offer. "I figured you could use some help if you want to make first string."

Manny looked up the stairs that rose above them, back and forth, higher and higher. "How many floors?"

"Seventy-three."

"That's a lot."

Pete snorted dismissively. "Walter Payton used to take new Bears running backs to the 108-story Sears Tower to run up and down the stairs until they collapsed, puking up their guts."

"Tough guy."

"Hall-of-Fame tough. Payton strengthened his legs as a kid running up and down the sandy banks of the Pearl River in Mississippi in 100 degree heat and 99 percent humidity. In the Sears Tower, Payton was always the last back standing."

Manny nodded, craning his head back to eye the stairs that led up out of sight above them. Looking back down at Pete, he asked, "What's in the backpack?"

"Water bottles. Makes it a little harder for me; gives you a chance to keep up." Pete's record was doing all 73 floors twice before collapsing exhausted, but he hoped to better that record this fine morning, especially with some competition, of a sort. Pete intended to be the last linebacker standing at the team tryouts in August, regardless of what the hotshot transferring linebacker, Joe Cain had done in Texas.

"Let's go," Pete ordered. He led the way up the metal stairs two at a time, his footfalls reverberating in the concrete stairwell.

By 4 p.m. the day after Mr. Danny Molina stroked out on his way to the operating table, the Mount Hermon Significant Adverse Event Committee had convened to review Julie's study. The committee met whenever a clinical trial subject died or suffered a significant, unexpected health setback.

"Mr. Molina experienced a stroke four years ago," Julie said as she concluded her report on her patient's medical history. "His risk of another stroke was 25 percent."

"Why was he included in the trial?" her chair, Andrew Baxter asked, flipping through a thick file folder filled with reports, forms and data from the study.

"We didn't think a history of stroke would be contraindicated for the trial," Julie said. "All the drugs we're using have been thoroughly tested and should not have been contraindicated for patients who had experienced a stroke."

"Tested alone, but not in the combination you're administering them, correct?" Baxter asked.

"True." Julie had hoped her chair would be more supportive.

"You appear to have some promising data, thus far," Steve Goldman, a rheumatologist, commented. Young, bright and ambitious, Julie respected and liked Steve. His wife was a doll; an ex-nurse and, unlike many of the women who married a doctor, far from focused on money and status.

"The data thus far are promising in the areas of memory, cognition and creativity," Julie agreed.

"But also a long and growing list of negative side effects," silver-haired Patricia Rhys-Jordan noted. She was dressed in designer clothes and, as always, looked camera-ready. A cardiologist with a nose for publicity, Rhys-Jordan, it was joked around the medical center, never conducted a study unless the results would make national headlines—and her studies always did.

"For the most part, not serious side effects and manageable with moderate intervention," Julie said, trying to sound optimistic as she defended her study.

"Any other patients at high risk for stroke?" Baxter asked.

"Mr. Molina was not at high risk," Julie shot back, and immediately regretted it.

Baxter started questioning her about how she had determined risk of stroke for each of the patients in her study. Then he switched to a long, involved series of questions about high blood pressure, osteoporosis and the other side effects the patients in the study were experiencing. The other committee members deferred to him, asking a few tangential questions, apparently because they felt as the neurosurgeon on the committee, the study fell within his area of expertise. The thought flashed through Julie's mind that this would be one of the few committees that did not count Rick Severn among its members; he'd support her.

Facing the possibility that her clinical trial would be cancelled, an attacking department chair, and a foot that throbbed after a day in the OR, in clinic and rounding that had started at 6:30 am, Julie knew her temper was short, but she also knew she had to remain calm and answer all Baxter's questions.

As they sparred Julie realized that Baxter had never even read the detailed study plan he had signed as chair of neurosurgery, even if his name as director of the laboratory would go on every abstract, article and patent application that arose from the research. She wondered why Baxter was leading the charge to question every detail of her study and realized that he was protecting himself. After Mr. Morris' death and, God forbid, if any other patients should die, Baxter wanted to ensure no one would have grounds to accuse him of being anything other than thorough and prudent in approving and then monitoring the study being conducted in his department. You did not become a department chair at a major medical center without playing politics as proficiently as the Medicis at the height of their power.

"I'm still unclear why you included such patients in your study," Baxter mused as if it was a comment about an appetizer on a menu.

"Most patients with Alzheimer's have extensive medical histories," Julie said, keeping the anger she felt out of her voice. "Finding a patient with AD and no other conditions is close to impossible."

"It does seem clear that the patient who expired was at high risk for stroke, with or without the trial drug regimen," the young rheumatologist Goldman said.

"Given your monitoring, I wouldn't be surprised if the incidence of stroke in your study is lower than the incidence in a similar sample of the patient population you drew from," the camera-ready Rhys-Jordan suggested.

Baxter sniffed, looked around the table and, seeing that no one else had a question or comment, said, "I think we have enough information to make a decision. If you'll please wait outside, Julie."

As she stood outside the closed double doors, Julie felt the tension caused by the stern questioning from Baxter ease from her body, replaced by worry over the fate of her study. She fidgeted as she debated whether to sneak outside for a quick cigarette. She had no idea how long the committee would deliberate and she was supposed to be quitting, so she stayed put.

Reviewing the meeting, she felt certain that the study would be allowed to continue. Baxter was against her, but Goldman, Rhys-Jordan and the others appeared to believe that the study should not be terminated. Many studies had lost a patient and continued, especially studies involving geriatric patients or the terminally ill.

Twenty worry-filled minutes later Julie walked in, her face set in a businesslike mask to hide the throbbing in her foot and the sliver of fear that her study would be canceled. Rhys-Jordan and Goldman smiled at her: a good sign. Her study would not be cancelled. Relief eased the tension in her body. As she sat down, her cell buzzed in her lab coat pocket. She glanced at the number: the ED.

"Excuse me, please, it's a patient-care call," she told the committee. Patient care trumped all other responsibilities.

"Julie, it's Patrick. Another of your study subjects is here."

"Presentation?" Julie asked, dreading the answer.

"TIA, possible stroke."

*Dictionary is the only place that success
comes before work. Hard work is the price we
must pay for success. I think you can
accomplish anything if you're willing to pay
the price.*

—Vince Lombardi

March

"Again?" Amanda asked, stretching the word out into a whine. "You already worked out this morning."

"I have to workout twice a day if I'm going to get a scholarship to a decent college program," Pete said. He slung his dark-green workout bag over his shoulder as he headed out the front door past the slim, coltish Amanda. He could smell her perfume; sweet, like melted clover honey. The Santa Ana winds were blowing, bringing with them hot, dry desert air that pushed the mercury up into the high 80s near the coast.

Amanda asked, "I thought you were going to try for a baseball scholarship?"

"I like football better."

"But baseball is a....nicer sport."

Pete shook his head.

"What about basketball?" Amanda asked. "It's more fun to watch."

Pete shrugged. "I'd rather play football."

In tight black shorts and a mid-riff baring white top, Amanda turned to follow him to his late model BMW. His two-door car had a gash in the driver's door from an unfortunate encounter with a post at his gym's parking lot. During one of her kicks to instill greater responsibility in him, his mom had said he would have to pay for the repair, but Pete never seemed to have the money to fix it. Whenever he got some money from odd jobs, a video on how to be a better linebacker, a new pair of sneakers or a concert ad caught his eye and the money was spent.

"I thought we were going to the beach today," Amanda said.

"We were, but you're late, so I can't now," Pete said, setting his bag in the trunk of his car, which was full of football pads, a helmet and scuffed footballs.

"I wasn't late," Amanda whined, sounding far younger than her 16 years.

"We said just after lunch. It's almost three."

"I haven't even had lunch yet." Amanda loved sleeping in.

"Want some *hamantaschen*?"

"What?" Amanda looked as if he had offered her broiled road-kill.

"Cakes my mom makes for Purim."

Amanda still looked lost.

"It's a Jewish holiday."

"Sounds boring."

"You get to eat little cakes and make lots of noise. I used to love it as a kid. Mom loves the cakes, so she still makes them."

"I think I'll pass on the hama-hama-whatever."

Pete opened his car door but, taking in the pained look on Amanda's pretty face and her filled-out top, said, "If we go to Huntington Beach, I can go."

"Why not Redondo?"

"Huntington has steeper dunes."

Amanda tilted her head in a pout. "You're not going to run up and down the dunes the whole time again until you stink with sweat, are you?"

Pete encircled her with his muscular, tanned arms, smelling her just-washed hair, and said, "I have to. Jayden's working out twice a day and there's a new guy transferring in from Texas; All-State linebacker. If I don't workout, I might not even make the team next fall."

"You'll make the team. Danny Doyle says you're a great tight end."

"Danny Boyle?" Boyle was a reporter for the student newspaper. What did he know about football? "I want to be a linebacker and, even if I wanted to be a tight end, college scouts say I have to play more than one position; I can't get cut as a linebacker."

"If you did, you could spend more time with me. I sometimes think you love football loads more than me."

"You'd still go out with me even if I wasn't on the team?" he asked with a wry grin.

Amanda glared up at him, aghast. "That was the rudest thing you've ever said to me." She broke free of his arms and turned away, lowering her head in a pout, her emerald eyes wet around the edges.

Pete sighed. "Amanda, I didn't mean it. It's just that football's important to me…"

"And I'm not?" she spat back.

"Of course you are, but I want to stay on the team, get into a good college and make the pros so we can have a great life together, like we've talked about."

"Like you've talked about."

"If I make it to the pros, we'll both be set for life. I'm doing this for both of us, Amanda." As he put his arms around her from behind and held her tight, feeling her firm body against his, the tension drained from her body. He could just feel the bottom of her breasts with the tops of his forearms. His lips close to her ear, he kissed her neck and whispered, "I do need to workout today."

Amanda broke free again and, stalking down the driveway toward her new black convertible, yelled back over her shoulder, "I think I'll pass. Robyn's going to the mall. I may as well go with her and Erin, and have some fun for a change rather than watch you sweat."

Pete took three strides toward his girlfriend's coupe, but the engine started and Amanda swerved out into the street and was gone. Pete swore, spun on his heel and stalked back to his car. He damn well better make the team or he wouldn't have a girlfriend, a football scholarship or a future.

Ah, a man's reach must exceed his grasp —
or what's a heaven for?

—Robert Browning

"I am sorry, but the committee ruled that it's in the best interests of the patients to discontinue the study," Julie explained to Mr. and Mrs. Croft in a Neurosurgical Institute clinic room. She could have had nurses call the study patients to tell them, but she would not delegate the onerous chore nor would she do it with a telephone call. It was a major decision to participate in a research study and she owed her patients; she would tell each one face-to-face. This was her nineteenth such conversation.

"But why?" Mr. Croft asked, his gray eyes slits as he struggled to comprehend the news.

"The risk was deemed to be too great."

"The risk of what?" Mr. Croft reminded Julie of a Leprechaun. He was frail with pale, parchment-like skin stretched over high cheekbones and a prominent chin. His eyes, while gray, often caught the light and sparkled a shade of blue she had never seen before.

Julie said, "One of the patients suffered a stroke and passed away."

"Not to sound callous, but they must have been old to be in the study in the first place. It isn't like Alzheimer's strikes the young."

"No, the patient was geriatric," Julie admitted, wishing the conversation was not heading down this path.

"Then the stroke probably had nothing to do with the study."

"That may be but he died, and a second patient suffered a TIA, a transient ischemic attack, which carries a one-in-four chance that the patient will suffer a stroke within five years."

"Five years? I don't know if I'll be alive let alone remember who I am in five years, drugs or no drugs." Mr. Croft looked down at his hands, flecked along the cuticles of the flat, square fingernails with oil paint in a rainbow of colors. "What's the life expectancy for Alzheimer's? You probably told me, but I can't remember."

"In general, it reduces your life expectancy by half," Julie explained, glancing over at Mrs. Croft, who took in the information with a remote look. Julie wondered if Mrs. Croft understood any of it or if she was just glad all the tests, drugs and paperwork associated with the trial were over—as well as Mr. Croft's painting hobby.

"What does that mean for me?" Mr. Croft stared unblinking at Julie.

"You have a life expectancy of about 20 years, so that means Alzheimer's would reduce that to about 10 years. I should add that there's great variation. Some patients your age might live 25 years, others far less than the average."

"Ten years or a risk of a stroke in five," Mr. Croft said, "I'd rather take the drugs and the risk."

"I'm sorry but I can't prescribe them to you." Julie had known this would be hard, but she was finding it more difficult than the conversations she had every day when she told patients they had a glioblastoma multiforme, astrocytoma or glioma and had only a few months to live. With those patients, she was just a messenger telling a patient something that had already happened to them. She was not responsible for their condition. With Mr. Croft, she was responsible. She was no messenger; she was an executioner. "It's out of my hands," she said. "I just can't give you the drugs."

"Why not?"

"It would be unethical."

Mr. Croft pursed his thin, white lips.

"It would be immoral," Julie said. "As a physician, I'm trained to do no harm, besides the fact that I could lose my job and my medical license."

Glancing at his wife who continued to clutch her handbag on her lap and stare in the general direction of Julie, Mr. Croft asked, "How long will the effects of the drugs last?"

"They should be out of your system in 24 hours, but the effects may last longer. To be honest, no one knows. That was one of the many things the study was investigating."

Leaning forward in one of the clinic room's hard, plastic chairs, which squeaked, Mr. Croft looked up into Julie's eyes, his brow furled. "So I'll lose my ability to paint soon?"

"I fear so, or at least whatever part of it came from the drugs."

"All of it." He blew the air out of his mouth in a long, slow, emotional sigh. His head lolled forward. Julie thought he might be crying, but then the white-maned head came up again and with clear eyes he asked, "Can't I keep taking the drugs? I could buy 'em from Canada or Britain or somewhere. I hear they sell such things over the computer these days."

"I'd strongly advise against it. They could kill you."

"I'll die anyway."

"You'll probably die much sooner on the drugs."

"Better dead than unable to paint."

"You could suffer a stroke that could leave you incapacitated and unable to do much of anything, let alone paint."

"With Alzheimer's I won't be able to do anything either, including paint. Can't you just let me keep painting? It's all I have."

Julie glanced at Mrs. Croft, but she sat there, nodding at what her husband had said, but with a glassy, bored look, as if she was waiting for a child to finish playing before taking him home.

"I can't."

"Can't or won't?"

"Both."

"If it was your dream, wouldn't you take the drugs?"

"I don't know, Mr. Croft."

"What's life without a dream?"

"Life."

When you are not practicing, remember,
someone somewhere is practicing,
and when you meet him, he will win.

—Ed Macauley, Hall of Fame basketball
player, b. 1928

April

Saturday was a good day to start things. Julie rose early, showered, dressed, checked her email and, having answered the important ones, deleted the junk and left a few to respond to later, set out for a jog. The punctures from the pit bull had closed and her foot was healed. If she was going to run the LA Marathon on May 25 she had to get serious about training—now.

Saturday was a good day to put things behind you. She decided as she loped along the path near the old Red Line, which had been a trolley line in the 1940s, that she would put her research on hold for a while. She would focus instead on operating, writing fiction, training for the marathon, and Pete. It would be nice to shift priorities for a while. She had been working 12-hour days for so long she couldn't remember what life was like without them.

Returning from her jog, her legs tight, her chest heaving, but feeling strong and refreshed, she drank a glass of cool water in the kitchen. She spotted a printout of an online bill from a florist. The brief note was to Amanda from Pete, asking her to forgive him.

Julie hoped it wasn't serious. He and Amanda seemed like a good match.

Julie went over to her purse. She took out a pack of cigarettes and with fierce determination threw them into the garbage can with a rewarding thunk.

"For good this time?" Pete asked as he came through the back door, returning from his morning run. His gray Spartans football T-shirt was dark with sweat. His long black shorts ended above thick, hair-covered legs and sneaker-clad size 11 feet.

"You should have told me you were jogging today," Julie said. "I would have gone with you."

"You go too slow."

"You go too fast."

"Ready for tomorrow?"

"Ready. I've missed football."

"For all of three months?"

"It was a long, boring three months."

"You played basketball and baseball."

With a predatory grin, Pete said, "There's no tackling in basketball or baseball."

It was Sunday morning and the dew still sparkled on the grass. The purple Jacarandas that lined the edge of the expansive park cast long, intricate shadows across the football field. Pete was in perfect position as the running back burst around the end of the offensive line. Pete hit the ball-carrier low and felt the impact as he slammed into the back's pads. His helmet reverberated as it crashed into a pad in the other player's football pants. No gain; a perfect defensive play.

The back spun, pumped his legs and drove up field. Pete fought to bring the back down to the turf. All he managed to do was cause the back to veer to the right instead of heading straight up field. The back gained precious yard after precious yard. Desperate to find solid footing as he was dragged along, Pete summoned all his strength to bring the back down. The back kept moving forward.

Finally Pete felt the back going down. Even as relief and triumph flooded his body, Pete realized that Jayden had sprinted all the way across the field from his weak-side position to assist on the tackle.

"This is spring football camp, Tomlinson, not a spring cotillion," yelled one of the college coaches who moonlighted running the camp for promising high-school players. "If you want to dance, choose a partner with nicer tits than Roberts."

"I'll dance with you anytime, Tomlinson," Roberts, the running back said inches from Pete's face as they lay entangled on the turf. "Dance your white ass all the way into the end zone."

"Screw you," Pete swore as the back bounced to his feet.

Frustrated and seething, Pete scrambled up and jogged back toward the huddle, muttering curses.

Coaches yelled, gestured and blew whistles as they worked their charges on the fields that made up Bruce A. Arnold Park. Some coaches worked with quarterbacks on perfecting their throwing techniques, others worked with linemen on blocking drills while still others put running backs through brutal running drills around cones and over ropes strung in squares a foot off the ground on rust-stained metal stakes.

"You need to add some muscle mass, Tomlinson, or they'll run over your ass all day," Jayden told Pete as they stood, taped hands on padded thighs, in the loose, defensive huddle. Even though it was early, sweat dripped off Jayden's tanned, hawk-like nose. Jayden gestured at a skinny safety. "Hell, Rodriguez, could tackle you with one hand."

"I work out every fucking day," Pete said, his frustration showing. He had never had this much trouble at a practice camp. He'd missed three tackles already and it wasn't even 9 am yet.

"Not hard enough," Jayden said.

"I work out hard."

"There's a difference between working hard and working smart. You have to use your head and I don't mean the tiny one between your legs. You work out the same way every day?"

"Yeah."

"There's your problem," Jayden said, earning glares from the other players who waited for him to make the call for their next defensive formation. "Work out a different set of muscles every day or all you're doing is destroying muscle."

"Let's go," a cornerback, Malthius, urged Jayden, expressing the resentful mood of the huddle at the delay.

"Fuck off," Jayden said with a dismissive grin, then added to Pete, "Read some stuff on biomechanics or you're just wasting your time sweating every day in the gym. Okay, red-five-six, and Malthius, try and cover your receiver this time instead of giving him a five-yard cushion. My grandmother could catch the ball if you gave her that much room."

Give sorrow words;
the grief that does not speak
Whispers the o'er-fraught heart,
and bids it break.

—Shakespeare

Julie was returning from a six-mile run before breakfast when she spotted Alan McGhee, part-time pit-bull-wrangler, struggling to get out of his red, two-door sedan in his driveway, just down from her house. He was using metal crutches. She veered across the quiet magnolia- and jacaranda-lined residential street to help, but by the time she arrived he was standing by his car, having steadied himself. He had even managed to maneuver a black backpack out of the backseat.

"Good morning," she said as she came to a stop behind him, jogging in place to stay loose. She debated whether to run another mile, but leaned toward not doing so, given the time.

He wore black shorts with a gold patch on the left leg with a black knight's helmet and words beneath the helmet in gold that she could not make out.

"Oh, no," she said, noticing a post-operative brace on his right knee as he shifted his pack to his other hand. She stopped jogging in place. "Please don't tell me you wrecked your knee rescuing me from that pit bull."

"No, no, no," he said, shaking his head and breaking into a smile. "I had a scheduled surgery last Friday. It had nothing to do with the pit bull."

"Oh, I'm so relieved. Well, not that you had surgery, but…."

"I understand."

Julie fell silent. She was talking too much and too fast. Her heart was racing—from running?—and she felt nervous and excited and happy, all at the same time. What was happening?

"Can I help you inside?" she asked, slowing her words as she gestured at his backpack, which he held in one hand by a strap while he handled the crutches.

"I'm getting better with these things," he said, wiggling one of the matte silver crutches in the air, "but I could use some help, if you have the time?"

"Of course."

She took the backpack, which felt as if it was full of books, and walked along beside him as he settled onto the crutches and hobbled around his car.

"How did you injure your knee?" she asked, even as she told herself not to ask too many personal questions.

"Just one of those things."

As they rounded the back of the car, she shifted the heavy backpack to get a better grip on it and her eyes fell on the license plate.

"A purple heart?" she asked, seeing the symbol for the medal on the left end of the California plate.

Alan stopped, glanced at the plate and turned back to face her with a look of chagrin. "My men got that for me. Wish they hadn't."

"For your knee?"

"For my knee, my hip, my eardrum and most of my right side."

"What happened?"

He hesitated, considering her with an appraising stare.

"If you don't want to talk about it, just say so and we can move on to other topics," Julie said hurriedly, "dog attacks, Bengal tiger sightings and my son's goal of gaining 20 pounds in the next three months."

"Why on earth would he want to do that?"

"Football."

"So much explained with just one word," Alan said with a knowing smile.

"Extremely parsimonious."

"Such big words for so early in the morning."

"Let's stick to simple ones then, like knee and injury."

He chuckled. "I was wounded in Afghanistan."

"I'm so sorry. What happened?"

"Wrong place, wrong time."

"I'm sure there was more to it than that."

A silence fell between them. A crow flew past overhead, casting a brief shadow over them. She met his eyes and said, "I've seen people in the ER who've been through some pretty horrible things."

"I tend to take the soldier's view that you should do what you have to do and then forget it."

"Some things can't be forgotten."

He dropped his gaze as he leaned on his crutches.

After a long moment, Julie said, "I'd like to know what happened, if you'd like to tell me."

After a long silence she was about to drop the subject, when he raised his eyes to look at her, managed a smile and said, "Would you like a coffee?"

Julie and Alan sat at a country-style, oval oak table in his kitchen sipping black coffee, his crutches leaning against the back of his straight-backed ladder chair. Macduff, having greeted Julie with a roar as if she was a long-lost littermate, had circled down onto an oversized and well-used tartan pillow in the corner nearest Alan's chair.

In the living room through which they had walked to reach the kitchen, Julie had noticed shadow boxes holding military decorations, including a Purple Heart, a Distinguished Service Cross, which made her pause, and several more she could not identify. There were photographs of young-looking soldiers—boys—with Alan in a tan and dusty land. The soldiers clustered close around Alan, as if he was a source of protection, succor and maybe even life itself.

Settled in the kitchen, Julie noticed the neat order of the house. The kitchen counters devoid of appliances. The fridge gleamed white. A bookcase she could see in the living room was filled with novels, political science textbooks and white Army manuals on three shelves and dust-free mementoes on the fourth shelf: a jade

Buddha, an ornamental Arab dagger, and a beer stein with an alpine scene etched on it.

"Coffee fine?"

"Excellent," Julie said, smiling to reassure him.

"You sure about this?"

"Certain. I'm interested."

After a few long moments he began, his voice low, even and controlled. "We were in Afghanistan near the Tribal Areas along the Pakistan border. An IED took out a Humvee in the column I was commanding." He stared down at his coffee. "They used to put IEDs in dog carcasses or under piles of trash, but we started putting a few rounds into carcasses and avoiding piles of trash as best we could. The Taliban or Al Qaeda or both of them adapted. They learn fast; faster than we do. They're on the offensive, which is an advantage." He looked up at her, as if he was teaching a class and was waiting for her to take notes.

She nodded encouragement.

"They started hanging IEDs from trees or, in the cities, lamp standards. The one that hit the Humvee in my column was one of the first we ran into that was hanging from a tree out in the boondocks. They knew we'd come along the road because it was one of our MSRs."

Julie frowned.

"Main supply routes from Pakistan."

Julie nodded.

"Ironic, in a way."

"Why?"

"One of my lieutenants later wrote me that that evening our command center received intel about a change in Taliban tactics sent from a unit in the northwest, near Shir Khan."

"Let me guess; a change to hanging IEDs from trees?"

Alan nodded with a melancholy look. He swallowed, rotated his coffee cup emblazoned with "US Ranger" a couple of times and said, as if he could see it happening before his eyes, "The explosion peeled the armored Humvee's roof back in every direction like one of those old bags of Jiffy Pop."

"The top isn't armored?"

Alan shook his head. "If anything, the armored sides concentrated the blast inside the vehicle. Killed two of my men."

"Oh, God," Julie whispered, wincing.

He stopped and stared at her. His eyes, dark and clear, seemed to search her soul. Appalled, shocked and feeling a sense of unreality at what he was saying in a quiet kitchen in West Los Angeles, she managed to say, "Go on," even as she tried to convince herself that the United States was at war: actually two wars.

"We established a defensive perimeter. I wanted to assess our casualties, and then move out to find and fix the bad guys. We'd been taught from Basic on to attack outward in an ambush. Seize the initiative and take the fight to the enemy, fast."

He rotated his coffee cup a few more times as he continued, "I heard some brass later figured out that such tactics never work. To catch the Taliban or the insurgents you have to lay an ambush at a likely IED spot or have patrols catch them setting the IEDs, which means a huge number of patrols. Way more than we could ever mount, although the surge helped." He paused to sip his coffee. He set the mug back down on the table, still cradled in his hands. "Tastes good. I used to chew on the grounds in Afghanistan to stay awake."

"As a doctor, I wouldn't recommend it."

"Gotta stay awake if you want to stay alive," Alan said, grinning. "No choice when there's no chance to boil water, although I prefer the liquid kind."

"I'm glad you choose the liquid kind this time."

"I went to see to my men. The two who were dead were in God's hands, but the driver had somehow survived. We called for medi-vac. Just as I finished the call and was about to order my men to expand our perimeter to go after the bad guys, the world fell in on us.

"They'd been waiting for us to form a perimeter around the destroyed Humvee. I was crouched beside the wounded man as the medic worked on him when an RPG—rocket propelled grenade—flashed over my head. Sounded like an F-16 making a low-level pass. Burned off some of my hair."

His hand went to the left side of his head, his fingers ruffling through his short hair as if following the track of the RPG's back-blast.

"They opened up with small-arms fire and mortars that must have been nearby. I could hear the clunk when each round dropped into the tube and the thump when it left the tube. The mortar crews had it all pre-sited. They walked rounds right along the ditch, where most of my men had taken up positions. It was the only cover in the area, so they knew we'd end up in it."

He paused, shut his eyes and opened them to look off through the kitchen's back window at the well-kept yard with its deep green grass, palms and fig tree.

"How did you get injured?" Julie asked after a few moments.

He looked back at her. "I didn't want to lose another soldier. I'd lost three on the tour already and two more that day. Most I've ever lost on a tour. No way was I going to lose another."

He turned his coffee another rotation.

"The rounds were kicking up the dirt on the gravel road around us and the burning Humvee was dinging like a music box as rounds struck it. Three of my men had managed to extricate most of the ammo for the fifty out of the Humvee, so at least those rounds didn't cook off."

"The fifty?"

"Fifty-caliber machine gun. There was one mounted on the roof of the Humvee before the IED blew it into a field half a click away."

Julie nodded, although she had no idea how far a click was.

"The medic and I dragged the wounded driver into the ditch. Although it looked deep enough to provide cover, it was sloped so the side away from the road left us exposed. The fire was so heavy, the medic and I squirmed out of our IBAs—body armor—so we could pile it over the driver until the helo arrived."

"Is that standard operating procedure?"

"His body armor was shredded by the IED—next to useless. He needed ours."

Alan glanced out the window and then back at Julie. "My troopers fought well. I sent a squad on a flanking movement around a rise to assault where I had fixed the mortars' location. We were doing pretty well. We were taking all they could dish out without suffering any more casualties save for a couple of shrapnel wounds. Then the Blackhawk came in. That's when every bad guy in the area opened up on it. They love to take down our choppers.

"The medic, another soldier and I lugged the wounded driver to the Blackhawk and got him aboard as a couple of Apaches came in and hosed the hill we were flanking with their mini-guns. We slid the driver into the chopper. I scraped up my left hand on the deck because I didn't get it out from under the driver fast enough; he was a big boy, 19 years old, but big."

Alan looked down at his left hand, flexing the fingers, even though any bruise or scrape had long since healed. "You know what?"

"What?" Julie whispered, fearful of intruding on his story.

"At that moment I thought I'd saved one of my men; saved him for his wife and kids and parents and friends and buddies. Saved him for birthday parties and anniversaries, promotions, new cars, drinking beer, watching movies, making love to his wife, and growing old with her, even if he hadn't met her yet. Last thing I remember is thinking: I saved one of my men."

He stopped.

"Then an RPG hit the Blackhawk."

He looked down, moved his coffee mug a quarter of an inch across the table and fell silent, motionless, his face blank.

Julie felt the silence in the kitchen. The whirr of the fridge intruded. The windows were closed, but she heard a car drive by outside. A bird chirped. Her coffee sat before her on the table, no longer steaming, the aroma dissipated.

"Did the Humvee driver survive?" she asked, her voice low, not wanting to know, fearful of the answer, yet needing to ask.

"No. The RPG hit the back of the chopper, I'm told. Pilot, copilot and the crewman on the Blackhawk survived, amazingly. With the chopper doors open, most of the blast went sideways, not forward. They had serious injuries, but I met them all at the hospital in Landstuhl. Thanked them. They did a fine job even landing in the firestorm the Taliban were throwing at us."

He stopped again, turning his coffee mug slowly, reverentially.

Julie waited, and waited, and then asked, her voice a whisper, "What happened to you?"

"They said I was blown back away from the chopper. Shrapnel from the RPG and the remains of the Blackhawk tore up my right side, mangled my knee, shredded my thigh, perforated my liver and spleen, gave me a concussion, broke three fingers and blew out my eardrums. Singed most of the hair off my head, too."

"You don't remember any of it?"

"Not a thing after I heard the whoosh of the RPG. I woke up on another Blackhawk, strapped down with a Medic working like a speed demon to keep me from bleeding out. My right side looked like I'd been stabbed with a serrated kitchen knife about 120 times."

Alan sipped his coffee. Setting the cup down, he glanced at his right side, moved his leg in its brace and added, "The medic, and the doctors and nurses at Landsuhl and Walter Reed did a wonderful job. You can barely see the scars now, except from where the biggest pieces of shrapnel hit me." His eyes drifted up over Julie's shoulder and out the window. "A wonderful job."

Julie suppressed a smile; patients always judged a surgeon by the scars they left behind.

After a few moments, Alan said, "I had to threaten the doctor to let me out of Walter Reed to attend Specialist Jason Michael Woodley's funeral in Elyria, Ohio; pretty little town, near the lake. Beautiful day with an honor guard, family and friends, some fellow soldiers, and the sun shining bright. Twenty-one years old." He stopped, shaking his head. "I went to five other funerals for my men: Specialist Giovanni Andrew Goldman of Queens, New York; First Lieutenant Stephen Kenneth Alonzo Washington of Wade, North Carolina; Lance Corporal Gregory Anthony Chu of Mendocino, California; Specialist William Jack Pearson of Pioneer, Wyoming; and Justin Romero of Olathe, Kansas."

His recitation complete, Julie waited for him to say something more, but he remained silent.

"People die in war," she said quietly.

"Yes, they do; young people. Wish I'd got that intel a little earlier. Wish I'd started my men attacking outward right away to clear those mortars."

"Would it have made a difference?"

"After two tours in Iraq and one in Afghanistan, you'd think I'd be better at it."

"They don't give Distinguished Service Crosses to incompetents—or cowards."

Alan looked at her, sizing her up, a slight frown creasing his forehead.

"My little brother loved military history growing up. I got to know all about insignia and decorations."

He nodded, moving his head slowly, as if moving it faster would shake the memories from his head. "Funny thing, when I woke up and found out what had happened, I was so thankful it was me waking up and that I hadn't been killed. I was so glad, so happy that someone else had been killed, not me. I felt damn horrible for thinking it, but I did—still do half the time."

Julie watched him, letting him talk, letting him move through his thoughts and emotions, slowly, with great difficulty as if he was pulling them out of his mind like anchors out of thick mud.

"After my tour in Iraq years ago, I wondered why I'd been riding in the Humvee I'd been in and not the one behind it that got shredded by an IED. Why wasn't I the one in the shower when a mortar round impacted and blew Chu apart on a stifling August morning? Why did Romero and Goldman get cut down by a machine gun when we were assaulting a hill near An Nasiriyah and not me, three feet to their left? Why was Washington killed by a sniper on a patrol in Baghdad like a dozen patrols we'd run before? And why was Pearson hit and killed by a prime mover carrying ice cream after he returned to base at 3 a.m. from a mission? It made no sense; no sense at all."

He glanced down at his coffee. "Now I know it isn't supposed to make sense. It's war. People die for no reason. People survive for no reason. All you can do is your best and pray every day. The guilt you feel, the sense of loss, the sense of futility, all of it's necessary. You can't avoid it, no matter how much you talk about it. Our society thinks guilt and sadness are bad, negative, but some of it can't be talked away. They're part of knowing who you are; part of being an officer, a soldier, a human being."

They sat for a time, each drinking their lukewarm coffee, the world passing around them. The fridge stopped whirring and a pair of hummingbirds buzzed at the window near where a glass feeder filled with red sugar water hung from the eaves.

"As a doctor, I lose patients," Julie said, trying not to sound as if she was minimizing what he had gone through or making any comparison at all. She wanted him to know who she was. "At first it tore me up inside. During my residency, when I lost a patient, I'd write my brother, sister or parents these long letters about death and dying; dark, somber letters. Made them wonder about my mental state.

"I thought I'd done something wrong if I lost a patient. I hadn't done enough. I didn't know enough. I had to learn more about glioblastoma multiforme, astrocytomas or whatever tumor, malformation, condition or disease had dared to kill one of my patients. It drove me to learn, to perfect my surgical skills, to check, double check and triple check every procedure, every treatment, every suture, every prescription. Everything had to be done right, every time."

She sipped her coffee. "But I learned that even if I did the best job I could do—the best job anyone could do—patients still die. The best neurosurgeon on earth loses patients. There's no way around it, except to stop being a surgeon. The better you are, the less likely it is to happen, but it will still happen. So you learn to compartmentalize your emotions. If you don't, you can't do your job. At some point, you have to accept death as the price of being a doctor." She stopped and looked across the table at him, meeting his dark eyes and added, "Or, I guess, an Army officer."

"You'd think I would have learned that by now, but I still want to bring the same number of men home that I brought over."

"That's what makes you a good officer. I'd like to save every patient I see, but I have to deal with people dying every day."

"Every day?" Alan looked aghast.

"Every day I see patients from MVAs—motor vehicle accidents—who are brain dead, strokes incapacitate people to one degree or another, tumors, arteriovenous malformations and all manner of other conditions leave patients so close to death they may as well be dead. I see patients who aren't themselves any more and never will be. It's part of my job to talk to families about their loved one and try to get them to decide what should be done—or not done—to extend their love one's life."

"Sounds horrible."

Julie pursed her lips and nodded. "I love operating, taking someone who can't see into the OR and rolling them out two hours later with a tumor resected and their vision restored. In a way, nothing's better than operating on a baby with hydrocephalus. Before the procedure the baby arches their back in pain, screams non-stop and is near death. Forty-five minutes later, I've relieved the pressure on the brain and the baby is smiling and happy with an excellent chance of leading a long happy life. Best of all, the look on the faces of the parents makes you feel as if you've given them a piece of Heaven back and, thinking of Pete, I probably have."

"Even in Iraq during the worst of it, I didn't lose people every day."

"Everyone dies, somewhere, somehow—and a lot of them die in a hospital."

"Better to die on a battlefield fighting for something; at least if you die, it's for a reason."

"Reason or not, it's still a death."

Once you agree upon the price you and your
family must pay for success, it enables you to
ignore the minor hurts, the opponent's
pressure, and the temporary failures.

—Vince Lombardi

"I never thought I'd see the day," Julie announced late Wednesday night as she walked into Pete's room and found him cradling a textbook the size of the Oxford English Dictionary. She saw glossy medical illustrations on the page he was reading, which stood in stark contrast to the Bears jersey he wore. "I thought you were going to be a football player, not a doctor—or maybe a football-playing doctor?"

"Nope, just a football player."

Julie glanced over at Pete's bookcase. Long ago the few books on the shelves—mostly how-to-play football and biographies of famous players—had been pushed back to make room for football trophies and game balls. At one time he had loved to read. What had happened?

"What's this?" Julie asked, fingering a supple black leather jacket that hung from the back of Pete's desk chair.

"Just a jacket I got."

"Bought?"

Pete nodded.

Julie sighed. "With what?"

"Some cash I had."

"From where?"

Silence.

"You know you're not supposed to gamble."

"I haven't been."

Julie looked down at her son, reading his face. It had been so much easier to tell when he was lying years before. Now he barely seemed to care whether she believed him or not and, oddly, it made it impossible to tell if he was lying. "I hope you haven't been."

He turned a page.

Resigned to pursuing the gambling issue another day when she had more energy, Julie sat next to Pete on the faded Chicago Bear's blanket that covered his bed and had since he was 12. "What are you reading?"

"Biomechanics."

"Excuse me?"

"Biomechanics, it's the study of..."

"I know what biomechanics is." Julie suppressed a laugh. "May I ask why?"

"I heard that if you work out every other day you build a lot more muscle than working out every day. I want to know if it's true."

"I think that's right, but I'm far from an expert on biomechanics."

"Even if you do know what it is?" Pete asked with a mischievous grin.

"You're still not gaining enough weight?"

"Nope," he admitted, regret and anger in his voice. His blunt, thick index finger traced along as he read, pausing, Julie noticed, at some of the longer words.

"It can take a long time to build muscle," Julie warned.

"It's already April, four months until tryouts and I've barely added a pound since the end of the season."

"Certainly not for lack of trying."

"Jayden's already put on seven pounds."

"Some people just gain muscle faster than others."

"If I don't put on some weight soon I'm not even going to make the practice squad, let alone the first string, especially with this new linebacker coming from Texas."

Julie had never heard Pete so negative. His usual confident determination seemed to be failing him. "You're one of the top linebackers and tight ends. I'm sure you'll make the team, at least as a tight end."

"I want to be a linebacker. What does atrophy mean?"

"It means that something withers or weakens." Julie looked at the text. There were a lot of specialized biomechanical words, some of which even Julie didn't know the meaning of. "Why don't you tell me what you want to know and I can do a little research at work. I know a couple of physiotherapists."

"Physio-whats?"

"Physiotherapists. They study movement and physical ability, usually to do with people recovering from an illness or broken bone, but also for athletes. I might be able to find some answers for you."

Pete kept reading, then with a sigh slammed the hardcover book shut and asked, "Tomorrow?"

"I'll see what I can find out."

"Tomorrow?"

"Yes, I promise, tomorrow."

"I want to know the best weight-training schedule to build muscle fast while not losing any flexibility or speed."

"Especially for football players?" Julie asked with a knowing smile.

"Especially for linebackers."

"Okay." She rose and headed for the bedroom door. "And tight ends?"

"Yes, but mostly for linebackers."

"Try and get some rest."

She walked back down the hall toward her bedroom. As she reached her bedroom door, he yelled, "Especially middle linebackers!"

Julie hesitated and then walked up the stone steps to Alan McGhee's glass and oak front door. Pausing, she stood up straighter to her full five-foot-seven-inch height and pushed the doorbell.

A moment later, Alan stood before her. Instantly she forgot her carefully planned words. Her mind filled with a rush of conflicting, confusing thoughts as he invited her into his living room. She handed over *The Life of Pi*, which he thanked her for. After stumbling through some pleasantries, which included confirming that her foot and his knee were healing well, she managed to say, "It's Passover in a couple of days."

"I'm still a little short on intel about the specifics of that particular holiday," Alan admitted.

She sat on the sofa. "Before Passover, you clean your house thoroughly, if you're Jewish." She glanced around his living room. "Not that you would need to."

"The Army only pays to ship a certain weight of personal gear to a new posting. It's a strong incentive to reduce to a minimum gear you tote around the world."

"I wish I could impose such a requirement on Pete," Julie said with a smile. She forged on, "Besides cleaning your home from top to bottom, you remove all prohibited food, called *chametz*."

"Such as Cuban cigars?"

"No," she laughed, "such as grains, bread, vinegar, alcohol, and cornstarch."

Alan appeared interested, but Julie hoped he wasn't just being polite. In any case, it was too late to turn back now.

"You collect the *chametz* and store it in a sealed off part of your house and you find a…a friend, a non-Jewish friend to sell it to."

Alan tilted his head to one side with a look of bemusement. "I'm not in the market for any cornstarch, but I could use a nice bottle of wine: something that'd go well with the barbequed chicken I'm marinating in the fridge."

"You don't actually get to eat or drink the *chametz*."

His expression turned into a frown. "Then why buy it?"

Julie shifted on the sofa and plunged on, "So God knows I don't own or possess any *chametz* during Passover. Finding a gentile to buy it is called *mechirah*. It's not as common as it used to be, but my parents used to do it, so I thought maybe, well…"

Alan nodded and with great solemnity said, "I'd be honored to buy your Passover contraband. Do we get to haggle over the price? I got pretty good at bargaining when I was stationed in Turkey."

When Julie returned home, Pete, who was watching a DVD of the 1986 Bears Super Bowl win over the Patriots as he lounged on the sofa in his basketball uniform, asked where she'd been.

"Asking Mr. McGhee to buy our *chametz*."

"Our what?"

"The foods we can't eat for Passover."

"We've never done that."

"Yes, we have," Julie said indignantly. "We go to a *seder* and we never eat food that rises during Passover."

"Yeah, but we never sell food to neighbors."

"It's called *mechirah*."

"I've never heard of it."

"Don't tell your grandparents that."

"Why do it now?"

"Because it's Passover," Julie said, exasperated, and spun on her heel to stalk into the kitchen to prepare dinner as she wondered how she'd raised such a Gentile.

"I can't eat that," Pete announced a few days after Passover as he emerged from his room, eyeing the BBQ turkey burgers and seasoned fries on the kitchen table.

"Why not?" Julie asked, weary after a long day in the OR, clinic and three exceedingly boring meetings about the neurosurgery website, residency program and research funding. Hell must be an endless series of meetings, with each meeting devoted to discussing what to discuss at the next meeting. At least Alan had stopped by after she returned from work. He had returned her *chametz* in exchange for the $20 he had 'paid' Julie for it.

"I can eat the burger," Pete said, "but not the fries."

"Are you an American?"

Pete frowned up at his mother as he sat down at the table.

"Every real American loves French fries."

"I have to eat 40 percent carbs, 40 percent protein and 20 percent good fats to add muscle," Pete recited, ignoring his mom's exasperation.

"You don't even sound like a teenager any more."

"That info you got for me said I should eat…"

"I know, I know," Julie interrupted as she set the plate of burgers beside the basket of fries and sat at the table. Maybe she needed a cigarette or some wine, lots of wine.

"I need some brown rice and broccoli or green beans," Pete said.

"There's the kitchen," Julie said, pointing good-naturedly. "Vegetables in the crisper, as well as some frozen. Rice is in the cupboard by the telephone—brown and white. Cook all you want."

Much to her surprise, Pete bounded up and she soon heard him rattling pots, pans and dishes in the kitchen. With a sigh, she rose, covered the burgers and fries with napkins to keep them warm for her to eat later, and went to help him create his chosen muscle-building dinner.

Literature nowadays is a trade....
your successful man of letters is your skillful
tradesman. He thinks first and foremost of the
markets...

—George Gissing, English novelist,
1857-1903

Julie was sprawled back on her desert-tan sofa, laptop on her thighs in her quiet home. Although it was a warm night, a fire in the hearth threw shadows across the room. She was finishing a final proofread of a short story as the hands on the clock on the end table approached 11 p.m. She had surgery in the morning but she had learned as far back as medical school to subsist on far less sleep than the human body was designed to require. With Pete asleep, late evenings were a perfect time to write—at least on nights when she wasn't on call.

She scrolled back to the first page. She read the date on the top left corner of the title page. It had been a little more than four years since she had tapped out the first word of the story. Since then it had been written, revised, rewritten, submitted to a dozen literary journals, rejected, revised, rewritten, submitted to ten more journals, rejected, revised, and the cycle repeated again and again and again like some literary Sisyphean torture. The cycle could only end when the story was published or she gave up, and the later was unthinkable. Julie never gave up. With stout determination, she told herself that maybe this time the cycle would end. Someone would accept the story and publish it—only her third fiction publication.

Then and only then, she would succeed in pushing the boulder over the summit of the mountain.

She leaned back and gazed into the fire, listening to its crackle as the flames consumed a piece of bark, spitting embers against the fireplace screen. She stretched her neck and shoulders and thought for the hundredth time that she should write at her desk, not on her sofa. The problem was that proofreading a story felt more natural on the sofa: feet up under a plush throw, pillow under her head, sunk down in the deep embrace of the sofa cushions as if she was in a lover's arms. There was something different about reading a story more like a normal person, as a reader would read a story, drawing upon the creative, imaginative part of her brain, which was more willing to be immersed in the world created in the story. When she sat at her desk, back straight, feet on the floor, she drew from the more analytic part of her brain. In that position she tended to focus far more on the technical aspects of the story—specific words, grammar and spelling—instead of immersing herself in the story itself to try to decide if it was worth a damn as a story. From her reading of stacks of books on how to write and hundreds of novels from English classics to the most recent thrillers, she knew you could write a novel or short story that was perfect in terms of technique and grammar, yet if the story itself was weak, there was no hope of publication. If you told a rip-roaring story, the writing itself could be far from great, even pedestrian, and it would sell.

Taking a deep breath, she decided that her baby was once more ready to send out into the world. Opening another computer file, she proofread the email cover letter that would offer her story to the *Cimarron Review, Alaska Quarterly, Comstock Review* and seven other literary magazines and journals across North America. She had a list of 296 fiction markets as far away as England, India and Hong Kong on her computer, as well as a sub-list of 10 journals for each story she was working on and for every story that was out. She kept the lists ready so that when a rejection arrived, she already knew where she would send the rejected story—after she had read and revised it once, twice or thrice more. It helped keep the depression brought on by rejection at bay, at least a little, preventing it from enveloping her in its dark embrace for more than a day or two after a rejection arrived. A college boyfriend who had majored in psychology had commented that creative writing was the longest un-reinforced behavior known to man or woman. From painful experience, Julie had to agree.

An hour later, the cover letter perfected and the short hand on the clock past the 12, she used the blind email function to submit the story to all 10 journals. Some did not accept simultaneous submissions, but after 15 years of submitting dozens of short stories to journals and having published just two, Julie could see no harm in speeding up the process. If she didn't, it could take years to submit a story to 10 journals, since many took six months to reply. The odds of anyone wanting her story, let alone two journals wanting it at the same time were so insignificant that she was more than willing to run the risk of having to explain to one journal why she was publishing in another journal a story she had submitted to them. She dreamed of such demand for her stories.

Supposing you have tried and failed again and again, you may have a fresh start any moment you choose, for this thing we call 'failure' is not the falling down, but the staying down.

—Mary Pickford, Canadian movie star, co-founder United Artists, and of the Academy of Motion Picture Arts and Sciences, 1892-1979

Morning sun cascaded through his bedroom window as Pete, naked, stalked into his bathroom. Staring down at the scales, he debated whether to cheat a little and weigh himself after breakfast. No, that would prove nothing. He always weighed himself before breakfast.

He had been working out, eating right, devoting himself to getting bigger and stronger in the manner prescribed by the notes his mom had taken after talking to a physiotherapist who specialized in sports medicine at Mount Hermon. It had to pay off. He flipped open the black binder on the bathroom counter in which he kept track of his daily weight. He tried not to linger on the depressing sameness of the figures on the damp-rippled white pages. He had gained four pounds since the end of football season in December. Four pounds could be water gain for all he knew. Maybe today would be different.

He stepped on the scales, looked down and waited as the red indicator coursed across the electronic screen once, then twice, before it displayed the number. Wincing, Pete looked up at the ceiling and let out an anguished groan.

With the advent of email submissions, literary journals were getting faster with their rejections—or at least the first round of outright rejections. Within two weeks only one journal had not responded—negatively—to Julie's short story submission. Then it did: "Thank you for your submission, but our editorial board has decided that your story is not suitable for our journal. We receive thousands of submissions every month and regret we cannot provide individualized feedback. Literary judgment is subjective, so please do not take this decision as a reflection on the merit of your submission. Even though your story is not right for our journal, we hope it finds an appropriate home elsewhere. Best wishes."

Julie thought she must be getting worse as a writer. She had received more form rejections this time than ever before and faster than ever before, whether for a short story or a novel. Wondering what she could be doing wrong, she considered taking more creative writing courses at UCLA Extension. She had taken a dozen over the years. They had varied in their quality depending on the instructor. A few teachers just told everyone their writing was good or even great and made few suggestions about how to improve. A few instructors were far better. More critical, they made dozens of valuable suggestions for each story she submitted. After taking the courses, reading stacks of how-to books and writing a few million words, she had felt that she had improved. She had been receiving longer, less form letters of rejection and had even received a few letters asking to see other things she had written. Best of all, she had published two short stories in reputable literary journals.

Recently, however, she just got form rejections again. Had she hit her peak as a writer and then deteriorated? She had no way of knowing. Who could she ask? Everyone would have an opinion, but no single opinion would tell her whether her novels would ever find a market. One opinion—even an editor's—meant little. There might be a thousand, ten thousand or even a hundred thousand others who would love her work, if only they got a chance to read it. Editors were the key to allowing people a chance to read her novels, but even experts found it difficult to recognize greatness in literature. The list of Nobel Prize winners in literature was far from a consistent list of literary greats. For every Kipling, Yeats and Faulkner, there was a Frederic Mistral, Henry Sienkiewicz or

Gerhart Hauptmann. Of the roughly 100 writers who had won the prize, Julie recalled recognizing only about 35 when she perused the list, and the vast majority of the 35 had been in the past 20 years, when she'd heard the media coverage about the announcement of the prize. At best, one in 20 winners was remembered or read much, if at all, after their death. The record of the Pulitzer Prize was no better. Who had ever heard of Julia Peterkin, Oliver LaFarge or Margaret Ayer Barnes? If expert committees established to reward the finest writers failed at recognizing lasting greatness, how good could one editor be at some obscure literary journal? Unfortunately, posterity chose great novelists from those who had been published, not from those who had not.

Even among those who published and sold well, most failed to find lasting greatness. Dickens, Byron, Twain and Shakespeare did well in their lifetime and were famous long after their death, but such a relationship between popularity and greatness was far from assured. Julie recalled reading a book by Frank Luther Mott, who had studied bestselling American novels. He found that few bestsellers survived beyond their initial popularity. For every *The Call of the Wild*, there were a dozen bestsellers that no one today had ever have heard of, such as Gene Stratton Porter's *Freckles*, Alice Hegan Rice's *Mrs. Wiggs of the Cabbage Patch* and George Barr McCutcheon's *Graustark*. Popular fiction rarely became lasting literature.

The reverse also occurred. Some writers never enjoyed publication, let alone success when they lived, yet were recognized as great after they died. Although he had success with his early novels, Herman Melville was assailed for his later works, with one review not only questioning his greatness, but his sanity, stating in its title, "Herman Melville Crazy." After failing to find a publisher for his first novel, John Kennedy Toole committed suicide in 1969. His mother then found a publisher for *A Confederacy of Dunces*, which won the 1981 Pulitzer Prize for Fiction. Julie had read that Swedish investigative journalist Stieg Larsson died of a heart attack at age 50 in 2004 leaving behind three unpublished novel manuscripts, which were published posthumously to great success. In 2004, Chilean poet and novelist Roberto Bolaño died of liver disease at the age of 50. In 2009, his last book, *2666*, appeared in the United States and Britain to rave reviews and staggering sales. Unfortunately, Julie had no way of knowing if her novels and stories would be hailed as great after her death. In any case, she preferred knowing whether she was any good as a writer while she was alive rather than hoping for posthumous success.

Sighing, Julie wished she had been born without the gene that drove her to write—if there was such a gene, and if there wasn't, she wished her environment had never molded her to dream of becoming a novelist. She recalled Faulkner's quote, "The worst habit anyone can form is writing. You can form other bad habits and you can cure yourself, but you can never cure yourself of writing." Maybe she should switch from researching Alzheimer's disease to determining how to treat the disease that drove people to write fiction. The cumulative decrease in pain and suffering if she was able to cure people of the desire to write fiction, she thought with a wry grin, would be roughly equal to the cumulative decrease in pain and suffering if she cured Alzheimer's, besides ridding the world of a dozen library's worth of badly written fiction. Julie just prayed that her fiction did not fall into that category.

*In the 1972 Munich Olympics, American
Steve Genter swam in the 200-meter freestyle
days after surgery to repair a collapsed lung.
The stitches opened and Genter lost a pint
and a half of blood as he swam without
painkillers since they violated Olympic rules.
He lost to Mark Spitz by .95 of a second.*

At a weekend football camp, Pete reached the front of the line for a blocking drill. He faced a running back who had to be 20 pounds heavier than he was—all of it muscle. The power back's shoulders were wider than Pete's. His muscular thighs and calves bulged through his tight white football pants. Even his neck, barely showing between the scuffed and scarred helmet and the jersey-shrouded, flat shoulder pads, was corded with muscle.

Seeing Manny Ortiz, the skinny, sophomore safety behind the power back, Pete wished he had been facing Manny instead. Steeling himself, Pete got set. His body tensed.

"Hike!" the linebacker coach barked.

Pete and the back hurtled into each other. Before he knew what happened Pete was on his back on the grass, gasping. He fought to draw air into his lungs. Nothing happened. Terror spread through his body as he lay on the ground, fighting for air. His lungs had collapsed. He couldn't get any air. He was dying.

He panicked as he struggled to get his diaphragm working. His eyes widened as the linebacker coach, a former Oakland Raider linebacker, hauled him to his feet like a toddler. The coach encircled him with his burly arms in a bear hug. Pete's terrified mind thought the ex-Raider had lost his mind. Had the coach decided to crush him since he couldn't even execute a decent tackle?

Pete felt a quick, intense squeeze. Air rushed back into his lungs.

"Thanks," Pete gasped to the coach, his body relaxing as oxygen flooded into his grateful lungs. The terror that he couldn't breathe passed, leaving him with a glaze of cold sweat all over his body.

"You betta get some pounds on you son or learn to play with the wind knocked outta you," the muscular coach said in a rich Southern drawl. "Now get your ass back in line and try it again."

Pete sat slumped on a wood bench in the locker room at the school hosting the football camp. The cracked and stained concrete floor was littered with tangled balls of white adhesive bandages, empty clear plastic water bottles, grass, dirt, and, here and there, drops of dried blood. All the other players had left for the day. Pete had showered and changed into his street clothes, including his treasured Bears jersey and beloved leather Santa Maria High team jacket with the white patches for making All City, All State and for the team reaching the city championships two years in a row, but he lacked the energy to get up and drive home; not only the physical energy, but the emotional energy to bother. He had never had such a poor practice. Backs had run over him. He and Jayden were known as the finest line-backing pair in the state, if not the country, but today Pete felt far from being anywhere near the best on the field, let alone the state.

"Pete?" It was Coach Paukenan. The broad-shouldered, sandy-haired ex-Wisconsin quarterback sauntered into the empty locker room and sat beside Pete, his long legs straddling the slats of the graffiti-covered, nicked and battered bench. "I've been watching you out there."

Pete nodded. Paukenan often came to watch his players at the various spring football camps run by college coaches and ex-pro players across Los Angeles. Paukenan liked to get a jump on determining who would make the team in the fall and who would not.

"You're having some trouble with the bigger running backs," Paukenan observed, "especially the power backs."

Pete said nothing, still staring at the concrete between his sneakers.

"As a tight end, you still block well, but when you have the ball you're being taken down by cornerbacks and safeties. A tight end should be able to run right over them or at least drag them five yards."

Pete nodded.

"There's a new linebacker, Joe Cain, transferring from Texas this fall." Coach said it conversationally, as if only mentioning it in passing.

"I heard, coach." Pete wished he were somewhere else, anywhere else.

"He's All State."

"I'm All State." Pete looked over at the tanned, taut face of his coach.

"Football's competitive in Texas; lot of fine players."

Pete nodded. Football's competitive in California, too.

The coach ran an index finger over his thin lips, ruffling his clipped, blond moustache. "I've always been straight with my players, so I'll be straight with you."

Pete knew and dreaded what was coming. He wanted to sprint out of the locker room. He didn't want to hear it, but he had no choice.

"I'm sorry because you did a fine job for us last year, but watching you out there, I can see that you're not getting the job done. As it stands now, Jayden and the new boy from Texas, Joe Cain, are my first picks for our two linebacker slots. You know my defensive scheme only uses two linebackers on most plays, so if you want to make the first squad next fall, you need to work harder, put on some muscle and show me you can stop the bigger backs."

Pete wanted to scream that he was working harder than he ever had, that he worked harder than Jayden, harder than anyone on the team. He was in the weight room before Jayden and left after him. He ate right. He'd seen Jayden downing burgers and fries, pizzas and sodas, and drinking enough beer to float an aircraft carrier. Pete ate fruit, vegetables and a balanced diet that was supposed to build muscle quickly according to expert physiotherapists. He drank one beer at the most and never smoked. He worked on his speed with Adina. He studied biomechanics to make sure he was moving right, tackling correctly and training as effectively as he could. What else was he supposed to do? What more could he do?

Pete realized the coach was staring at him, waiting for a reply.

"I'll do my best, Coach," Pete managed to mumble amid the roaring emotions that engulfed his brain.

"Cain also put up some impressive numbers as a tight end." Coach left the implication clear. "Just wanted to let you know," Paukenan said with a forced, closed-mouth smile. "At camp in August, I'll look at all three of you with a fair eye—I promise you that—but right now, I'd say you need to get some work done to make the team. Understood?"

"Yes, sir," Pete said and forced himself to add, "Thanks, Coach."

Paukenan rose, put a hand on Pete's shoulder, squeezed it sympathecially, and then strode out of the locker room.

Pete's head fell into his hands. Frustration, anger and humiliation flooded his body. He had worked so hard and now his future, the future he, his father and even Amanda and his mother had dreamed of for years was about to be destroyed. No more Friday night games under the lights before everyone he knew. No more being recognized for being a great linebacker, for making a key tackle, for winning a game; no more, never again.

He would lose Amanda, despite what she had said. His mother, father and everyone who knew him would be shocked and dismayed at his failure. There would be no college, no NFL, no career. Nothing. Nothing left at all. He was 17 years old and his life was about to be over. Everyone he had ever told he was going to play college ball and then in the NFL would know he was a failure; everyone. It all boiled down to one word that would define his life and who he was: FAILURE.

He remembered the pride in his father's voice and even his mom's when he overheard them at family gatherings or parties talking about his success on the football field. The words that had made him glow with pride now just served to darken his mood and depress his thoughts even more.

Groaning, Pete wondered what the odds were that Joe Cain would break a leg or tear an ACL before he made it to California; just a little injury that would take him out for the season or even just a few games. Pete only needed a few games to show coach that he could—with or without more muscle—take down opposing backs, even power backs. In a game, Pete knew, fired with adrenaline and as focused as he was during games, he could take down any back. A practice drill at a camp was one thing; a real game was something else entirely.

But, he realized as melancholia flooded his mind, an injury to Joe Cain or Pete gaining the muscle by the start of the football season to take down stronger, bigger backs were both about as likely as his mom winning the Nobel Prize for Literature—her secret dream she had once confided to him. Both were about as long a long shot as the Browns winning the Superbowl.

"You seen Jayden?"

Pete looked over at Mike Lowe, who peered from behind a curtain of long black hair through the open doorway. Pete was surprised to see the science geek at a football camp, let alone in the locker room.

"He left," Pete barked, returning his gaze to the floor to stew and ruminate over his demolished dream.

"Ah, damn it," Mike said. He glanced outside, then slipped into the locker room, the door clicking shut behind him. "You're Pete Tomlinson, right?"

"Yeah." Pete sounded far from friendly, but Mike kept coming toward him.

"You're one of Jayden's friends, aren't you?"

"Sure," Pete said without enthusiasm.

"Can you do me a favor?"

Pete remained silent; what the hell did the geek want?

"I was supposed to give Jayden something, but I got tied up waiting in line for tickets to see Matchbox Twenty. Can you give it to him?"

"I'm not your delivery boy."

"I don't have time to go to his house. I have a date tonight and I'm already running late."

"A date?" Pete asked in disbelief, his curiosity drawing him out of his depression. Did science geeks date?

"With Jane Fraser."

"She's on the volleyball team," Pete said, frowning. Jane was hot. "How do you know her?"

"Tutored her in math. You'll see Jayden tomorrow at camp, so can you just give him this?" Mike held out a brown Manila envelope that bulged in the middle.

"What is it?"

"Just something he needs." Mike moved the envelope closer to Pete's hands. It rattled when he moved it.

"What's in it?"

Mike hesitated. "You're tight with Jayden, right?"

"Sure." Pete wanted to know what was in the envelope.

"You know what's in it," Mike said, his eyes narrowing and his lips pursing conspiratorially.

Pete considered. Curiosity won out and he snatched the envelope from Mike's hand.

"Thanks, Pete. Thanks a million."

Pete looked down at the sealed envelope and on impulse tore it open in one swift motion.

"Hey, what the Hell you doing?" Mike yelled. He reached for the envelope but pulled his hand back when he saw Pete's menacing glare.

"Just seeing what I'm delivering." Pete upended the envelope and out tumbled a bottle of pills. He frowned. "Steroids?"

"They gave them to Jayden for his knee."

"It healed a year ago. He can't still be taking them."

"Christ, you didn't know." Mike spun around, his black hair swishing across in front of his face. "God damn, Jayden's gonna kill me. Fuckin' roid rage. He'll tear my head off." He pushed his hair away from in front of his face and lodged it behind his silver-stud adorned right ear. "Jesus, I thought everyone on the team took 'roids."

Pete knew about steroids, but was shocked that Jayden was taking them. Mike reached for the pills. Pete put a hand on his chest and held them out of his reach.

Mike pleaded, "Don't say anything, alright? I'll take them over to his house. We'll forget all about it. Please don't tell him I gave them to you, alright?"

Pete stared down at the pills, still holding them away from the slim Mike.

"Come on, it's nothing to you."

Pete stared at the pills, his mind racing along the tracks toward what those white octagonal pills meant and what they explained.

Mike stood silent and then asked, desperation in his voice, "You want any?"

"Screw-up my body?"

"Make your body, you mean. You've seen Jayden. His knee is better than it ever was, and he didn't get that body by lifting weights and living right. Modern pharmaceuticals are the ticket to the pros."

"No thanks. Why do you sell this shit?"

"Engineering at the Ivy League costs money. I've got enough for freshman and sophomore years. I'm working on my junior year. Pays a lot better than Burger King and it helps the team; can't compete on the field today without the help of modern science."

Thoughtful, Pete slid the bottle back into the envelope.

"If you don't tell Jayden I screwed up, you can have a sample, free," Mike said, slipping into his salesman mode. "Put on some muscle; make pumping iron a lot more effective. I won't tell anyone, I promise." Mike dug a second bottle out of his pocket and held them out to Pete. "Give them a try."

One has no talent. I have no talent.
It's just a question of working,
of being willing to put in the time.

—Graham Greene, English writer, 1904-1991

May

In her office at Mount Hermon, Julie was boxing up the files from her terminated clinical trial when she stopped at Mr. Croft's thick folder. She flipped it open and leafed through the pages of notes and reports, stopping at the creativity tests. A graph showed little change in the pre-test period, but once he started taking the trial drugs creativity shot up with amazing speed. Julie traced the graph with her index finger from bottom left where it meandered along the bottom of the graph until the drug regimen began and the graph rose in a jagged, yet determined fashion toward the top right of the page. With a sad smile of loss, she closed the file.

"Sorry about the study," Baxter said, framed by her office's open doorway.

"Thanks," Julie said, struggling to keep the glumness out of her voice.

"You could try a different drug combination."

The scientist in Julie wanted to say that the original combination had been based on the results of several hundred studies conducted by thousands of researchers around the world. You didn't just switch the combination as if you were adding raisins to your blintz recipe. Researchers were supposed to devise a theory from which they developed hypotheses that could be tested. You were not supposed to just try different drug combinations for no reason until luck led you to an effective treatment. If you did, you would never know why something worked, making it next to impossible to build on what was known, let alone to know when to prescribe such treatments. Unfortunately that was how science was often done in these days of committees, publish or perish, and obscenely high payoffs from drug companies for treatments for common diseases.

"Well, come by and see me sometime if you want to talk about it," Baxter offered with an encouraging smile. "I'm late for a Board meeting."

Baxter was always late for one meeting or another. Did he ever operate any more? He did, she knew, but always with another neurosurgeon, usually the newest member of the Institute, who didn't mind losing half their surgical income to the director, even if he just poked his head into the OR for a few minutes to check what they were doing to justify his half of the bill. She knew she was being unfair given how hard he had worked to become director, but she would never forgive him for leading the charge against her study at the SAE investigation.

She realized that over the past few years her relationship with Baxter had been changing. Where once she had respected and liked him, she no longer did. It was hard to retain respect for, let alone continue to like, a boss who didn't back you up. Rick Severn had once said Baxter hated to share the limelight. Whenever any of the surgeons or researchers at the Institute gained a little fame, fortune or notoriety, Baxter dedicated himself to taking them down a notch. She doubted Baxter was even aware he did it.

"Lunch?"

Julie looked up and saw Severn slouched in her office doorway. She smiled and asked, "With who?"

"Me, of course." He returned her smile with an even broader one.

"Who else?"

Severn chuckled. "Am I so predictable?"

"Afraid so."

He lowered his head and, looking up at her, said, "You know me too well. Two reps…"

"Female reps, I'm sure."

Severn glanced down the hall behind him in both directions and, his voice low, said, "Actually they sent a rather striking brunette with a fine pair of legs and, get this, some guy. So, I thought, well…."

"You'd set me up?"

"What can it hurt? Good-looking young man, somewhat more mature, beautiful female neurosurgeon, why not?"

Julie chuckled, noted the compliment, but shook her head. "Why are they so interested in you?"

"Their company sells intra-operative MRIs."

"I'll bet my left arm that you dutifully serve on the committee deciding which new iMRI to purchase."

"You get to keep your arm. Use it to come raise a fork at lunch, please."

"I really can't."

"Why not?"

"Busy, busy, busy: surgery, research, clinic, training residents, committees, and a few dozen other little things."

"I heard your clinical trial got the kybosh. You must have some free time."

"Not really, but thanks for the invitation."

"Dr. Stein, you've got to learn to live life at some point," Severn said with mock seriousness. "This isn't a dress rehearsal; as far as we know this is your one shot at life. Grab your dreams, pursue beauty and make the most of it."

"Three wives and all?" Julie asked with a sweet smile.

"Touché, my dear, but you've only had one husband, so get with the program."

Julie laughed as her colleague sauntered off down the hall, whistling "When You Wish Upon a Star."

If she was taking a break from research and not going out for lunch with young medical equipment reps, she could write more. Even as she leafed through a Manila file folder she kept full of story and novel ideas, her mind rebelled at the futility of it all. As she sorted through the scribbled notes on slips of paper from pads she kept at her bedside, in her car, office, lab and lab coat, she struggled to stave off the frustration and depression that seeped around her like a dark, many tentacled beast, seeking to insinuate its hope-draining tentacles into her soul.

She had been writing stories and novels since she was 10. Over the years, agents and publishers had read her novels and even liked a few. Some had written encouraging letters of rejection, blaming their negative response on a tough market, a topic that "just won't sell right now" or an inability to place whatever novel genre she had submitted. For all the occasional words of praise, a "complex character," an "intricate plot" or "compelling dialogue," none had ever liked one of her novels enough to represent one, let alone to find a publisher. Futility thy name is creative writing.

Julie rose from her desk and wandered over to the window to peer out at the hospital's South Tower. Maybe she should quit writing. She had tried quitting twice before. Buried by 100-hour work weeks, neurosurgery had supplanted writing during medical school, her residency and fellowship, and then again a few years later when she landed her first position and had to build her practice. But as soon as there had been a sliver of a moment she could steal from medicine, her mind raced back to stories she wanted to tell, words she wanted to put down on paper, and characters she wanted to bring to life in print. Even as a senior resident she had written stories during some of the less challenging rotations.

Her mind had been split between neurosurgery and writing. The split had never been even, with the desire to be a novelist taking prime of place until late in high school when she'd realized that becoming a successful novelist was as difficult as becoming not only a doctor, but a Nobel Prize-winning physician. There are more than 200,000 doctors in the United States, but only a few dozen full-time novelists. Money was far from everything, but she wanted to be comfortable, and respected. Saying you were in medical school was far more prestigious than saying you were studying creative writing. So in high school she turned to science and discovered she was good at it. Medical school followed and medicine took precedence, even though writing still held sway over her soul.

She had desperately wanted to be a neurosurgeon, but that yearning was nothing compared to her quest to be a writer. The desire to be a novelist was always there, burning beneath the surface like an ember in her gut that, regardless of how frustrated and depressed she became about it, never burned out. Oh, how she wished and prayed it would burn out.

Once she accomplished her goal of becoming a neurosurgeon, she had thought becoming a novelist would be easier. Becoming a neurosurgeon had been far from easy. She had been the only woman in her class to choose neurosurgery, the only female neurosurgical resident, and the only woman she knew to pursue a doctorate to learn how to conduct research into the conditions that affected the body's most important organ: the brain.

If becoming a neurosurgeon had been hard, she reasoned, could becoming a novelist be any more difficult? At first, she had believed that becoming a novelist had to be easier than becoming a neurosurgeon. She had met mediocre neurosurgeons, but they were still far more competent at their profession than the writers who penned the bland, predictable novels with illogical plots, cardboard characters and wooden dialogue that she perused from bookstore shelves or the bedsides of patients. If you could be that bad and publish a novel, she should be able to publish a dozen novels—or at least she had thought so.

She had hoped that being a doctor would impress agents and editors. Maybe it had, but not enough to publish her novels. One agent had even called to ask for a second opinion about whether to stent or coil an AVM. After hearing her free medical advice, he didn't even offer any constructive criticism of her novel.

Now, years later, having succeeded as a neurosurgeon, the desire to be a novelist burned even brighter in her than before. Every time she was praised for her success as a neurosurgeon, she wanted to scream that it meant less and less to her; she wanted to be something else entirely. Didn't anyone realize that she was meant to be a novelist? Were they that obtuse? Did no one really know her?

When she stepped back to look at it objectively, she told herself that she had succeeded as a neurosurgeon because there was a defined path to that goal: college, medical school, internship, residency, fellowship, doctorate, and a position at a medical center. Then operate, do a good job, attract referrals, publish research, and keep working in the same research area, advancing your understanding of a single disease. Focusing on one condition also allowed her, like every other successful researcher, to publish papers rapidly, with each article reporting one incremental step in a broader research agenda. Ask any surgeon and they could tell you how to get to where they were. It was far from easy, but it was there, a well-trodden path ready to be followed, not to the top of the profession, but certainly well into the respected masses of a field.

No such path existed to become a novelist. Julie had spent years trying to discover where that path lay, but had found none. Some novelists had been to college, some had not. Of those who had, some studied English or creative writing, while others studied psychology, history, physics, or just about any other course of study offered at any university on the planet. Since she spent some of her time when she was frustrated and avoiding writing looking up the biographies of novelists on the Internet, she knew that writers such as Anton Chekhov, A.J. Cronin, Arthur Conan Doyle, W. Somerset Maugham, and, more recently, Michael Crichton had been physicians before becoming writers. But, physician or not, unlike medicine, there was no direct route to becoming a novelist. You had to write and write and write, and then, if you were skilled and lucky—Julie had no idea of the proportion of either required—someone published your novel.

She tried not to even consider the next step; the difficulty once published of selling more than a dozen books to your family and friends. She avoided thinking about the long odds that faced the first-time novelist, most of whom sold 120 copies and vanished into literary oblivion. The challenge of making a living by scribbling stories and selling them as novels was about as great as becoming not just a singer, but Pavarotti. Publishing in medical journals was far easier than publishing fiction. The prestigious *Journal of the American Medical Association*, the most widely distributed medical journal on earth, she knew, accepts eight percent of the more than 6,000 manuscripts it receives each year. Based on such acceptance rates, she had published more than 120 research papers. No fiction agent, let alone book publisher would ever even approach such an acceptance rate. A literary agent might select one new author a month, if not every six months to represent out of thousands of submissions while major book publishers do not even accept unagented submissions given the deluge of unsolicited queries they receive.

Whatever the degree of futility in continuing to write, Julie could not quit. When she did, she felt like a failure. She felt as if she was ignoring the reason why she had been put on earth. Raised religious, she had strayed, but not far. Religion was still in her, regardless of how much her scientific mind told her there was no empirical evidence of a divine being, let alone the odds of such a being conforming to human conceptions of him, her or it.

She still believed in God. Her image of him was of an elderly, bearded man who met you after you died. He sat on a wood stool behind a high, David Copperfield-era clerk's desk. Apparently Heaven had yet to enter the digital age. God ran his gnarled fingers down columns in a foot-thick ledger and found your name, "Julie Leah Stein." He ran his finger across the parchment columns and read, "Ah, yes, I gave you a fine mind for science and writing, great ambition, optimism, but with a slight depressive streak, some addictive tendencies to cigarettes, I see, a tendency to put on a little weight. Some running ability for distance, but none for sprints. Bit of a weak left knee, a spot of pneumonia as a child. So," he would say, resting his bearded chin in his weathered hand, "what did you do with what I gave you?"

She had a good answer for the scientific mind she had been given; "I became a neurosurgeon. I helped thousands of people: eased suffering, helped extend lives and when required helped ease the pain of death. My research too, if it continues"— it would continue after this unfortunate hiatus—"could benefit hundreds of thousands of people who suffer from Alzheimer's and other degenerative mental diseases."

God would nod and, leaning forward across his desk, would ask, "And what about your affinity for writing?"

Julie would have no answer save for a weak, "I tried."

In the image she had, she saw God staring down at her over his massive, dusty ledger with a look that betrayed that he thought she had far from tried hard enough. Everyone said they tried, the key question was how hard?

With a sigh she turned back to her cherry desk, drumming her fingers on the beveled edge and then leafing through the file folder of novel and story ideas: some good, some bad, most hard to tell if they would be great or garbage. You never knew how an idea would translate into a story until you wrote it, so how to choose which one to start writing? Worse, it took months to even draft a novel. It was not like writing a short story, a song or a poem. A wrong novel topic choice could waste a year or even longer. What to write, what to write?

Giving up was no answer; she could not. If she did, she knew that she would be doomed to wonder whether, if she had just kept trying, she might have become a great novelist. Was she a future Chekhov, Dickens, Twain, Hardy or Hemingway? Maybe her next novel would be the one that got published, the first stone in a path stretching out to literary immortality—or at least to a nice body of work of which she could be proud, even if few people ever read them. A body of work she would be able to show God when he asked the question she dreaded most.

Pushing thoughts of writing from her mind, she sighed and picked up a file from her desk. It was a drug inventory. Drugs for her canceled study. It would be best to send the drugs over to the pharmacy but, knowing Mount Hermon, there would be enough paperwork to wallpaper Cleveland to authorize the transfer of drugs from a clinical trial to inpatient use.

She sighed, using the file to fan her face. The air conditioning never kept up with the sun as it beat down on the row of windows in her southwest-facing office.

Increased creativity.

She stopped fanning, opened the file and stared at the list of drugs from her clinical trial. She looked over at Mr. Croft's painting on her wall. Rather good for a man who had never been trained to paint; for someone with Alzheimer's—incredible.

She looked back down at the list of drugs.

Every act of creation is first of all
an act of destruction.

—Picasso

As Julie pondered the drug list, the case of British novelist Iris Murdoch leapt into her mind from her research into creativity in relation to Alzheimer's. Murdoch had published her 26th novel in 1995, *Jackson's Dilemma*. Reviewers savaged it, even though Murdoch was a top writer, having won the prestigious Man Booker Prize. Murdoch later admitted grappling with writer's block while working on the novel; an early sign of Alzheimer's. Two years later, Murdoch was diagnosed with the disease. A researcher later compared Murdoch's first novels to her later ones and found a marked decline in sophistication. Patients with Alzheimer's struggle to express their thoughts, especially abstract thoughts, and use a shrunken vocabulary, which resulted in more pedestrian word choices by the once-gifted Murdoch as the disease progressed.

Julie leaned back in her chair. The drug combination she had prescribed to the Alzheimer's patients in her trial decreased the senile plaques in their brains and stabilized their brain cells' calcium balance. These changes appeared to restore creativity by reversing the decline in the ability to think abstractly and the loss of vocabulary and other cognitive functions related to creativity.

What would happen if a healthy person took the drug combination? Would they increase creativity or were the drugs merely reversing damage caused by Alzheimer's and returning patients to their pre-Alzheimer's creativity levels? That is what Julie would have guessed, yet there was the case of Mr. Croft. According to his wife, he had barely painted before being stricken by Alzheimer's, yet while taking the drugs he had become a decent, even good painter.

Julie knew that the majority of her trial subjects had performed better on creativity tests after they had been on the drug cocktail compared to before taking the drugs. The problem was that she had no way of determining how creative the subjects were before they fell ill. To test the drugs' effect on creativity, she would need to measure each subject's creativity when they were healthy, then wait years for some of the subjects to get Alzheimer's, and retest them with the disease and then again while they were on the drug regimen.

Julie sighed. She didn't want to wait decades to complete such a study.

"That sounded as melancholy as a dog who just lost a favorite bone," Rick Severn said from her office doorway, having returned from his free lunch.

"Just wondering why so many questions in science have too many variables and too little data," Julie said.

"And the human brain structured in such a way as to be far from bright enough to analyze it all most of the time," Severn said, coming into the office, a slim black tote under his tanned arm.

"Maybe someone else has come up with an answer," Julie mused, pulling her computer keyboard out on its tray from beneath her desk.

"Oh, goodie," Severn said, sitting down across from Julie.

Julie's eyebrows rose at Severn's choice of words, which didn't seem appropriate for a neurosurgeon in his forties, and his assumption that she wanted company.

Severn slid a gleaming red laptop out of the black tote. "I just got this new Mac and I want to give it a test spin. What are we researching?"

Julie couldn't suppress a grin as she took in Severn's eager, expectant face. "It's related to my Alzheimer's study."

"Yes," Severn said, leaning forward in his chair, hands on keyboard.

Julie pursed her lips and, seeing nothing wrong with letting Severn help her—as long as she didn't mention the real reason for her interest—posed the question, "Can drugs increase creativity?"

"Intriguing," Severn exclaimed, his fingers flying over his laptop's glossy red keyboard. "I love this stage of research; brainstorming, thinking, analyzing, and developing hypotheses to test."

Julie turned to her own computer and started typing. Using online journal databases that Mount Hermon subscribed to, she dove into the subject.

"'Drugs and Creativity: A Negative Relationship'," Severn read off his screen as he shook his head. "Doesn't look good for the hypothesis that drug treatment increases creativity."

"A lot of artists disagree."

"Artists?" Severn said with disdain. "I thought this was a scientific inquiry."

"A doctor should start with the patient, and artists are the most creative patients we have."

Severn looked far from convinced.

"William Blake," Julie read from a website. "English poet and painter."

"I've never had him as a patient, have I? I swear I would have introduced you if he had been."

"He wrote in the early 19th Century."

"Not one of mine, then."

"He wrote, 'The road of excess leads to the palace of wisdom,' and Arthur Rimbaud, a 19th Century French poet, said, 'The Poet makes himself a seer by a...derangement of all the senses.' Seems to support the idea that drugs enhance creativity."

"I just remembered one from my college days," Severn said, looking up from his laptop at the ceiling. "Baudelaire—a French poet; not one of my patients, either—advised, 'Be drunk always.' Advice I follow diligently."

"When did you ever memorize French poetry?"

"A master's in French literature at the Sorbonne before med school. Mom thought I should broaden my education. Dad thought it'd help me pick up chicks."

Julie laughed and, finding another website with information about alcohol and artists, reported that Edgar Allen Poe, Dylan Thomas, Evelyn Waugh, F. Scott Fitzgerald, Ernest Hemingway, James Joyce, Dorothy Parker, Eugene O'Neill, Jack Kerouac, and many other writers were famous for their epic drinking, as were artists Edvard Munch of *The Scream* fame and abstract expressionist painter Jackson Pollack.

Julie read off the site, "Five of the eight American writers who have won the Nobel Prize for Literature suffered from severe alcohol abuse or dependence."

"Then lets get drunk and write some literature."

"Hold the bottle. 'Although such great writers did go on binges'," Julie read, "'they were resolutely sober when they wrote.'" She shuddered to think what drivel would appear on her computer screen if she tried to write when she was hammered. Reading further, she found that writers who drank to excess produced their finest works when they were young. As drinking—and age?—took its effect, the quality and quantity of their work plummeted. As Beat writer Jack Kerouac concluded, "Drinking heavily, you abandon people, and they abandon you—and you abandon yourself—it's a form of partial self-murder." It also murdered the quality of a writer's work.

"Here's a study," Severn announced. "Gustafson and Norlander found that people drink more alcohol after hard creative work than after non-creative work, which might explain the image of the hard-drinking artist—but only after the writing is done." His eyes scanned the article on his laptop. "Drinking may be an attempt to alleviate tension caused by the creative process, which often unearths unconscious material that can cause internal conflicts."

"If you're writing about murder, betrayal or blackmail, and such things are drawn from your own life, exaggerated for effect," Julie said, "no wonder a writer could use a stiff belt after a day of digging deep into their deepest, darkest fears, hopes and desires."

"True," Severn agreed. "Says here that Eugene O'Neill's *Long Day's Journey into Night* was a retelling of the saga of his own family's bouts with drinking, success and failure. O'Neill's wife reported that he would often emerge from his study after a hard day of writing *Long Day's Journey* in tears, emotionally spent and exhausted."

"Lowe found that although moderate doses of alcohol had no significant effect on performance on a creativity test, there was significant individual variation," Julie said, having found another study. She hoped that alcohol might increase the creativity of those with an artistic inclination, but her hopes were dashed as she read on. "'Those above average in creativity who drank alcohol suffered a decrease in creativity while those below average in creativity showed significant increases in imagination under the influence of some alcohol.'"

Julie hoped she was above average in creativity or she'd never be a writer, alcohol aided or not.

"Maybe a stronger drug than alcohol is required to boost creativity," Severn suggested as he surfed on.

Julie considered the possibility and started another search. "Englishman Thomas De Quincey wrote a famous 1821 essay, 'Confessions of an English Opium-Eater' and Keats wrote in 'Ode to Melancholy,' 'My heart aches, and a drowsy numbness pains / My sense, as though of hemlock I had drunk / Or emptied some dull opiate to the drains.'"

"Sounds like they thought drugs were the way to go, but two subjects do not a clinical study make."

"Coleridge felt the same way," Julie said, having found a site about Samuel Taylor Coleridge and his story of writing his great poem *Kubla Khan* after awakening from a laudanum-induced sleep. Laudanum was a form of opium. Coleridge claimed that he composed "two or three hundred lines" of the immortal poem in his head as he slumbered. Julie wondered about the level of talent necessary to write a poem in your sleep that was still being read 200 years later. She would be overjoyed to write something when she was awake that was still read two years later.

According to Coleridge, when he awoke, he wrote the first 50 lines of the poem down and was about to write the rest when he was "called out by a person on business." By the time his business was done, Coleridge reported that he'd forgotten the rest of the poem.

"Should have strangled the 'person,'" Severn said, with unexpected vehemence, adding, "Read it in high school and loved it."

"Don't kill anybody just yet," Julie said, reading on. "Critics claim that *Kubla Khan*, far from being the fragmentary beginning of a poem, has a beginning, middle and end, which goes against Coleridge's claim that it was just the beginning of a poem he'd dreamed. Coleridge was famous for talking about poems or parts of poems he was about to write. The drug-induced dream story might have been nothing more than an attempt at creating 'buzz' for his poem."

"No need to find any laudanum for your Alzheimer's patients, then," Severn said. "Don't know if the stuff is legal anymore, anyway. Bunch of rock musicians swore by LSD, but apart from the vivid dreams, there's no evidence it enhances creativity."

Twenty minute later, Julie and Severn had concluded that the major difficulty research has found with drugs is that although individuals under the influence of drugs or alcohol may perceive things differently and be more creative, they are far from interested in sitting down to write a song or a poem, let alone penning a 300-page novel. Drugs decrease both the motivation to write and the cognitive ability to write well, and motivation is key. Poet James Russell Lowell wrote, "Creativity is not the finding of a thing, but the making something out of it after it is found." Drugs might help you find a creative insight but, once found, you're unlikely to be able to do anything with it.

Severn reported, "Norlander found that modest alcohol consumption helps in some stages of creativity, such as thinking of ideas, helping to overcome writer's block, lowering inhibitions, and delving into emotional subjects. The problem is that even moderate alcohol consumption detracts from other aspects of creativity, mostly the secondary processes, including preparation, the doing of the task, and judging the value of what is being done."

"Probably why there's the myth about the positive effect of drugs and alcohol on creativity," Julie said. "The use of alcohol and drugs make individuals believe they've performed better than they have after a project is completed."

"No one ever thinks they failed a sobriety test."

With a wry smile, Julie thought that if she started drinking, at least she would think she was a great writer.

"Moderate alcohol use at best has a negligible effect on creativity while excessive use has a negative effect," Severn concluded. "Marijuana produces similar findings, with little effect on creativity or cognitive abilities found in the short term, but harm being done to both faculties with long-term use. That explains the short careers of artists who use a pharmacy's worth of drugs on a daily basis."

Severn glanced at his simple, black watch and exclaimed, "Must be off." He shut down his laptop, clicked it shut and slid it into the black tote bag. "Committee meeting about the new intraoperative MRI machine we're buying." He rushed out the door, calling over his shoulder, "It's been fun."

Julie shook her head over her enthusiastic colleague as she returned alone to her computer search. She found one intriguing finding; researchers in 2001, analyzing the contents of clay pipes dating to around the time of Shakespeare in Stratford upon Avon, found traces of cocaine and hallucinogenic drugs. *Cannabis sativa*, the plant from which marijuana is derived, was available in Elizabethan England, as was cocaine. The researchers didn't claim that any of the pipes came from Shakespeare himself, but some scholars argue that some of his writing did refer to drugs. Sonnet 76 refers to a "noted weed" and "compounds strange," while in Sonnet 27 the Bard writes of "a journey in his head." Others scholars argue that a "noted weed" referred to a style of dress at the time, while "compounds strange" referred to unusual word construction or compound words.

Although her literature review lacked promise, Julie still wondered. Maybe, just maybe, the right drug or combination of drugs had not yet been discovered. Before Scotsman Alexander Fleming discovered penicillin in 1928 and Australian Howard Walter Florey developed it into a drug, there were no antibiotics. Before Jonas Salk developed the polio vaccine in 1952, there was no vaccine against poliomyelitis. Before the combined oral contraceptive pill, "The Pill," was developed and first tested in 1960, there was no reliable form of birth control. Someone had to discover each one.

Julie looked back at the list of drugs for her clinical trial. Were they the combination that would unlock creativity? Would they unleash a torrent of new artistic geniuses on the world? Were future Coleridges, Shakespeares and Twains out there, waiting for just the right drug combination to unleash their potential? New Titians, Rembrandts and Monets? New Rodins, Mozarts and Michelangelos? A new da Vinci?

She would have loved to devise a clinical trial to test her hypothesis about the drug combination's possible effects on creativity, but after the SAEs of her previous trial, there was no Institutional Review Board in the country that would allow her to test the same drugs again. She considered testing the drugs on rats, but given that creativity resides in the more advanced parts of the human brain, she feared that a rat brain was far too different in structure to assume that any creativity changes in a rat brain brought on by the drug combination would affect a human brain the same way—assuming she could figure out a way to measure rat creativity.

With animal and human trials ruled out, there was only one way left to find out whether the drugs increased creativity.

It was a daunting decision. She knew the risks: a TIA, a stroke or even death. But the rewards could be fantastic, and not just for her. Such a safe drug combination could aid millions of people suffering from the soul-destroying ravages of Alzheimer's and other neurological diseases. She had to admit that the greatest reward would be one that was intensely personal: a great novel, her long-held dream fulfilled.

Like a military emblem her brother had once shown her displaying a skull and the words, "Or glory," Julie faced a simple choice: success or death?

*The elect sneer at popularity; they are
inclined even to assert that it is a proof of
mediocrity; but they forget that posterity
makes its choice not from among the unknown
writers of a period, but from among the
known. It may be that some great masterpiece
which deserves immortality has fallen still-
born from the press, but posterity will never
hear of it; it may be that posterity will scrap
all the best sellers of our day, but it is among
them that it must choose.*

—W. Somerset Maugham, *Cakes and Ale*, 1930

June

Julie arrived home to find a belated rejection letter in the mail from *The Klondike Review*, a journal she had submitted a story to more than a year before. She had received such long-delayed letters before. Publishing ran about as fast as a tree grew. She read, "Dear Ms. Stein, Having reviewed your manuscript, I fear that we will be unable to offer you publication. Having read your story, I found:" A series of boxes followed next to pre-printed comments. The boxes that had been checked with black ink included "Unconvincing, cardboard characters," "Predictable plot," and "Uninteresting, tired setting," with a handwritten note alongside stating, "second story today set in a hospital." Beneath the boxes was printed, "I strongly urge you to work far more on your craft before submitting another story for consideration to any literary magazine. Yours, Anne Whalen."

Julie's body tensed, the anger rising in her like a fierce creature. Holding the offending letter with a grip that turned her fingertips white, Julie wondered what God-given power Ms. Whalen possessed to decide what would be published, what people would read and who would become an author. In all probability she was just a minimum-wage or volunteer reader at the tiny journal that printed all of 100 copies in frozen Alaska. What did she know about writing? Alaska hadn't produced a decent writer since Jack London and he hadn't even been a native; barely spending a year in Alaska during the Klondike gold rush.

It was the worst rejection letter Julie had ever received. Staring down at the letter in disbelief, she reread it to make sure she had read what she thought she had read. She had.

She stalked into her home office, brought her laptop to life and navigated to her file of journal addresses. Finding *The Klondike Review*, she deleted the contact information. With a vengeful grin, she went to the Trash folder and deleted the contact information from there, ensuring that it would never again sully her computer.

Athletics lasts for such a short period of time.
It ends for people. But while it lasts, it creates
this make-believe world where normal rules
don't apply.

—H. G. Bissinger, *Friday Night Lights,* 1990

Pete pushed open one of the school's side doors. He felt good after a sweat-drenching workout, not to mention the $350 from a winning bet on a Dodgers game in his favorite jeans' pocket. He glanced over at the playing fields that stretched to a line of cypress trees in the distance. The fields were empty, save for a lone football player driving a blocking sled across one of the grass fields. The player cast a long shadow as the red-orange sun set. The pollution of Los Angeles often made for brilliantly colored sunsets: light by God, filtered by man.

Pete stopped and watched from afar as the player drove the sled toward the end zone. Pete heard the thud as the player slammed into the sled. Whoever it was, he made good time. When the sled reached the end zone, the player stopped, trotted in place for a minute shaking his legs and then trotted toward the back of the school. As the player approached, Pete tried to see who it was. Pete edged behind the brick corner of the building to hide just as he made out the words on the player's dark blue jersey: Heatherdale High. Joe Cain, the new linebacker. Pete's body tensed with hatred as Cain trotted up the stairs to the school's rear entrance that led to the locker room.

After the door slammed behind Cain, Pete wandered down toward the blocking sled. He glanced up at the school several times, but saw no one. He reached the sled and, looking back up at the school once more to make certain no one was watching, leaned into the sweat-stained padded arm and gave it a cautious shove. It didn't move.

Pete frowned. He should have been able to move a blocking sled with little effort. Usually a coach rode atop it to add some weight, but even then Pete could move one across the grass at a good clip.

Glancing around the dark-green pad with a white Spartan "S" emblazoned on it, Pete saw that Cain had stacked a dozen concrete blocks into the bottom of the metal sled. Pete bit his lip. Dropping his dark green, Spartans gym bag onto the turf, he set his feet, leaned into the sled's blocking pad and pushed. His side of the sled rose off the turf. The sled squeaked and groaned. Grunting, Pete shoved harder and the sled moved—an inch.

Pete swore and backed away from the sled. It settled back onto the grass with a thud and a rattke. Determined, he set his shoulder. His nose was assaulted by the smell of aged sweat from the pad. He shoved the sled again. Sweat broke out on his back as he pushed. His shoes cut into the turf. His high-tops slid on the grass, then caught. Chunks of sod shot loose from his exertions. He pushed harder. The sled moved another inch.

Puffing, Pete stopped. He glared at the sled as if it was a malevolent beast.

"Fuck," he snarled. He snatched up his bag and stalked across the grass field toward the path that led to a pedestrian bridge across the aqueduct and, three blocks farther on, home. As he walked, he told himself he had just worked out for two hours. His legs were tired. He was worn out. If he had been fresh he would have been able to shove that sled across the field as if it'd been on greased wheels. The more he told himself that, the more he almost came to believe it.

There is no royal road to learning;
no short cut to the acquirement of any art.

—Anthony Trollope, English novelist,
1815-1882

Julie stared down at the six little pills on the granite bathroom counter. They formed a tiny painter's palette of different colors and shapes. She knew the names of every one, the benefits, risks and contraindications. She had some idea about their effects when taken together, one of which was boosting creativity—she hoped. The risks? Manageable.

She paused.

No, the physician in her had to admit that the risks could be far worse than manageable. Her trial had ended long before she could know the risks. Worse, she was younger than her geriatric trial subjects. She was healthier and stronger, but the age difference also meant that her body had far longer to experience, compound and run any risks associated with the drugs. But—and she thought it was an enormous but—she would only take the drugs for a couple of months while she wrote a novel fast. If French detective writer Georges Simenon could lock himself in a hotel room to create his novels in brief, explosive outpourings, so could she. Then she could stop taking the drugs before the side effects worsened or the risk of stroke became significant—assuming there even was an increased risk of stroke for someone her age. She could sell the novel and get her foot in the door.

Once she published a novel with the extra little creative help of the drugs, a publisher would be far more likely to publish her next novel written without any drugs. She had talent, at least enough to publish once she was given a chance. That was all she needed: a crack in the edifice of publishing that had, thus far, shown only a cold, stark face. Just one chance: just one. She had to get past the overworked agents and readers at agencies who were deluged by hundreds of book queries a week. If agents and editors were like they were in the 1930s, when they had—and took—the time to nurture new writers, she wouldn't need to take the drugs. She just had to get past the Ms. Anne Whalens of the publishing world and their check boxes of criticisms and find an editor with a true literary soul who would recognize her potential, talent and drive to succeed as a novelist.

She promised herself that after publishing a novel with the aid of drugs, if she couldn't publish on the basis of her own talent, then she would quit writing. She would clearly lack the gift, and she detested the idea of relying on drugs to succeed. She had to succeed on her own merits, albeit with a little help at the start from modern pharmacology to overcome the unfair barriers to a newcomer to the writing field. Many people had a little help at the start of their careers. She heard that Frank Sinatra secured his first gigs with the help of friends in the Mafia; "Book Frank or I'll kill you." She heard from an agent patient once that Nicolas Cage got his start acting in a movie directed by his uncle, Francis Ford Coppola of *The Godfather* and *Apocalypse Now* fame. A businessman she knew had mentioned that Donald Trump's first project while he was still in college was revitalizing a 1,200-unit Cincinnati apartment complex for his father's company. Not a bad start for a college student. Later, few knew, let alone cared, that such people had a helping hand at the start of their careers.

Even so, staring down at the pills, Julie hesitated. She had been hesitating for a month. She knew that most people—her mother, sister and friends—would think she was insane. She was a respected, successful neurosurgeon with a steady and growing practice, excellent publication record and a prominent position at one of the top medical centers in the country, if not the world. She owned a spacious, three-bedroom home—well, at least part of it, since the bank owned the majority of it. She had a handsome, athletic son who, even if his grades could be better, tried hard and was a fine young man. She was also, save for a few creaky joints, a stiff neck on occasion, and a touch of asthma, healthy. Why risk it all?

To write.

That is what it all came down to: she wanted to be recognized as a writer. Something in her makeup drove her to be a novelist. As she had read in H. G. Wells' *The Outline of History*, she had "that pathetic desire so common among human beings, to astonish some strange and remote person by writing down something striking,…" She could not stop it, could not accept that maybe she wasn't good enough. She had to be a writer. Success in every other area of her life paled in comparison to her dream of becoming a novelist. If being a mother, neurosurgeon or winning a marathon were each a 9 or 10 on a 10-point scale of satisfaction, contentment and happiness, becoming a novelist represented a 50, at least. It was so far above anything else, it could not even be measured on the same scale.

She stared down at the pills. Her father would understand, if he could understand anything at all. She had no choice. She could just as easily have decided to let Pete die of some dread disease for which she had the cure. It was no decision at all. She popped the pills into her mouth and swallowed them with a decisive gulp of water.

Desperation is the raw material
of drastic change.

—William S. Burroughs, US author, 1914-1997

Pete rushed into the bathroom with two white, octagonal anabolic steroid pills in the palm of his right hand. He stared down at the pills. For just a month, what would it hurt? He had to bulk up. All his hard work thus far had produced little, if any effect. His future rested on football: a good senior year, a scholarship to a top college football program and after four—maybe even just three— good collegiate years, a pro contract. His dream fulfilled. He had dreamed of playing pro since he was as big as a football, and the dream had never waned. When he played, he was in heaven. Full of adrenaline, his body strong, he felt invincible.

He stared down at the pills. If he didn't bulk up, he'd lose his linebacker spot on the team. Coach Paukenan had almost won the City Championship with a two-linebacker set last year and there was no way Paukenan was going to change his defensive scheme to use three linebackers this year.

Pete would be lucky if coach let him play tight end on some plays; Cain probably would take over those duties as well. Pete might try playing tackle, but he was meant to be a linebacker. It was more than a feeling, he had the tackle record and game films to prove it.

Working out, training and eating right had made no difference to his muscle mass. Without some help, he would be cut. Then what? His grades were decent, but far from the honor roll, something which drove his mother to despair. He wasn't going to get into a top school with his grades and, even if he did, what would he study?

He stared down at the pills. He shouldn't do this. He had to do this. Damn it all. He had no choice. What was the use in thinking about it?

He popped the pills into his mouth, swigged some water and swallowed.

The informed soldier fights best.

—US Army Orientation Booklet,
World War II

July

As Julie jogged past Alan McGhee's house on her morning run, the thought that she had been avoiding him came unbidden to her mind. She had been avoiding him, not with any conscious thought, but with a subconscious belief that she had little in common with a soldier. What did soldiers know? They knew how to kill. Or do? They ordered other men to their deaths. Julie was devoted to saving lives, not ending them. What could they possibly have in common?

For weeks as she had sped past each morning, Alan's California bungalow with the purple bougainvillea draped over the front veranda had returned a blank stare, devoid of any sign of human life. But this morning she spotted Alan perusing the newspaper on his front slate steps, Macduff snuffing in the grass in the front yard on a long leather leash.

Not giving herself time to reconsider, Julie trotted up his flagstone walk. "Morning," she said, jogging in place. "I see the cast is off."

Macduff roared and strutted over to her, tail wagging, head erect. She crouched to scratch him under the chin and rub behind his ears.

"Good morning. Yes," Alan said, extending his stiff leg and flexing it with great care. "Still weak, but healing nicely. The physio's a Jihadist; seems to think I should have been able to dance out of her lair after the first session. Coffee?"

"No, thanks."

Having been greeted, Macduff went back to his investigation of some interesting odors in the grass.

Julie glanced at a book that sat beside Alan on the stone step. Frowning, she asked, "*Anna Karenina*? I would have thought you'd be reading about war and history and generals and battles."

"I get enough of that out of the reports and manuals I have to read. My psychologist suggested writing about my experiences in Afghanistan, so I decided to read some good writing to know what to shoot for."

"Psychologist?"

"Army makes you see one after each combat tour."

"Tolstoy's certainly a great choice to learn from."

"I took a Russian lit course when I was doing my doctorate, so I thought I'd start with the Russians. Then read some English 19th Century novelists and then the Americans—Hawthorne, Faulkner and Twain," he said, picking up the thick novel. "It's good. Slower paced than novels today, but the writing is excellent. You start reading and before you know it 50 pages have gone by and you barely realize you're reading a story."

"Your doctorate?" Julie's mind struggled to adapt her image of Alan as she learned more about him.

He lowered his head and said as if it was the last thing he wanted to admit, "I got a doctorate a while back. How was your jog? You're foot okay?"

"Almost healed. In what?"

Alan frowned.

"Your doctorate?"

"You heard that, huh?"

"Yes, I heard that you have a doctorate. In what?"

"International Relations."

"From where?"

He hesitated.

"Is it a government secret or is your degree from Southwest Wyoming Community Teachers and Farmers College?"

He laughed. "Yale."

"I'm impressed."

"Just a ticket to punch on the way up the Army ladder," he said with a self-deprecating grin. "Two years reading a book a day and studying the past."

"Two years?" Julie asked. Doctorates usually took six years.

"Army pays for two years, so you do it in two years. It'll give me the option to teach at a university if I don't make colonel."

"I'm sure you'll get promoted." Even as she said it, Julie realized she hadn't the faintest idea what the odds were of being promoted.

"The US Army has 17,000 majors and all of them want to be a lieutenant colonel; fewer than half make it."

"Doesn't sound too bad."

"Did half the people you went to medical school with get forced to retire after 17 years?"

"No, but—"

"If you aren't promoted, you're encouraged to find employment elsewhere."

Julie smiled and said, "I'm sure the North Koreans would love to hire an American major."

"Could have done that back in the 1800s, but not now. Bit of an increase in nationalism. Don't much like *kimchi* anyway."

"Maybe Tahiti's army?"

"Probably already have the major they need for their 50 men."

"Couldn't you just stay a major?"

"The Army's up or out. No room for officers hanging around in a grade too long. Too many people below you want your slot. I can't blame them. I want the slot of a lieutenant colonel above me, so he better move up or out."

"Don't they want all the officers they can find for Afghanistan and Iraq?"

"They have a shortage of captains and majors, but they're swimming in colonels and generals."

"All the more reason to stay a major," she said with a smile.

"Up or out is still strong institutionally; besides, I don't want to be a major forever."

She stretched her hamstrings on the first step and asked, "Where are you from?"

"My father was career Army, so all over; the Deep South, Germany a few tours, Italy once, Japan and South Korea a tour each."

"Sounds exciting."

"In some ways. What about you?"

"Born in New York. My family came out to San Diego when I was ten. U of Washington undergrad, Oxford scholarship for a year, U Chicago Medical School, residency at Mayo, and a fellowship at Yale before I joined Mount Hermon."

"Impressive."

"You?"

"West Point and then wherever the Army sent me. Where'd you live in New Haven?"

"In a damp, cold cave the owner called a bachelor apartment on Sylvan Avenue, near the medical center. You?"

"Palatial digs on Livingston; prepared me for the rigors of being a prisoner of war if I'm ever captured by the North Koreans."

"I mention again that they'd love to hire an American major."

"And I mention again, *kimchi* and a climate that makes New Haven in the winter seem balmy."

"I didn't know the army let you go to school."

"They encourage it, even require it now. If you want to make colonel, let alone general, you better have spent some time getting letters after your name in some field other than military science."

"What's next?"

"Depends on how fast this heals," he said, gesturing at his injured leg. "Maybe a stint at the Army War College."

"Where's that?"

"Carlisle Barracks, Pennsylvania. Or I heard about an opening at a new center at USC they're establishing jointly with the military that sounds interesting."

"Not back to Afghanistan, or Iraq?"

"I'll be on limited duty for a time. I may deploy back to Afghanistan or Iraq as a colonel in a year or two to lead a brigade, if I'm lucky, but a year working with the new center at USC will let me stay here in LA for a bit and get this knee healed."

"I hope you get to stay….for your knee."

*In 1972 George V. Higgins was christened
an "overnight success" when he published the
critically and popularly acclaimed novel,* The
Friends of Eddie Coyle. *He later destroyed
the 14 unpublished novels he had written over
the 17 years before he wrote his
overnight sensation.*

August

"Ready for tryouts Monday?" Manny Ortiz, the sophomore safety asked as he and Pete emerged from the school. They had just worked out and Pete was already beginning to sweat again in the afternoon heat.

"I'm ready," Pete vowed. He felt good; confident he could beat Joe Cain for the second linebacker spot. Since his talk with Coach Paukenan at the weekend football camp he'd turned everything around. He'd continued his daily regimen of weight lifting, running stairs or sand dunes, eating right, and focusing on bulking up while maintaining his speed and flexibility. In 10 weeks, with a little help from Mike's pills, he'd added 22 pounds of muscle. He felt far stronger yet, thanks to Adina, he hadn't lost a single second of speed. He had even got a second faster in the 40. For such a short sprint, a second was the same as cutting a minute off a mile. He was even catching the ball better as a tight end and felt certain he could run over most cornerbacks and safeties, and hold his own against opposing linebackers.

His muscles suffused with blood, feeling rock hard and invincible, Pete said goodbye to Manny, wishing him luck at the tryouts, and drove his black BMW with the dented door to Amanda's house. They had patched things up after another argument over Pete's neglect of her; at least enough for her to accept his invitation to the party that night.

"What happened to your face?" Amanda demanded when he appeared on her doorstep.

"Nothing," Pete said, wondering what she was talking about as he felt his face with his hands.

"You can't go to the party looking like that."

She led him into the bathroom off her bright yellow bedroom. He peered at his face in the oval mirror over the pedestal sink. Acne had broken out all across his face, under his eyes, near the base of his nose, and across his forehead. It looked like an advanced case of leprosy. He had noticed some of it that morning, but it had rapidly spread and worsened.

Amanda opened the mirrored medicine cabinet and took out cotton pads and a bottle. She wet a cotton pad with the bottle's contents and wiped his face.

"Hold still."

"It stings."

"Toughen up."

Pete grimaced and tried to think of something else. "I got tickets to Linkin' Park."

"I thought you didn't want to go."

"I saw the tickets online and thought what the hell?"

Amanda applied dabs of ointment from a tube his face. The tip of her tongue protruded between her pursed lips as she concentrated on her ministrations. He reached around her to draw her close. Her pink top was just tight enough to provide ample evidence of the shape of her wonderful breasts.

"Stop that," she ordered. He let her go. "Clean your face with this twice day and then once a day put this cream on all the zits on your face," she instructed. "Should keep you looking nice and kissable."

"Thanks," Pete said, giving her a kiss.

"And avoid junk food; looks like you've been eating a bag of chips a day and bathing in olive oil every night."

"I don't eat any; gotta stick to the training regimen."

"Must be something else then."

Since she wanted to be on the clinical trial's drugs for the shortest possible time, Julie wrote every spare moment she wasn't sleeping, operating, in clinic, dictating, or attending this or that required meeting at the medical center. At first she started revising a short story, then, bursting with ideas, she started a new story before deciding to embark on writing the novel she had always wanted to write. It was to be a sweeping, intergenerational saga about a family with monumental dreams, yet only intermittent and moderate success, set against the major events of the past 100 years in America.

What once would have daunted her—plotting, character development, themes, research, and even the writing—the drug cocktail turned into a joyous endeavor. She had never been so excited, creative and bursting with great expectations in her life. Ideas poured out of her. She took a legal pad and pen with her in the car so she could jot down ideas as they flooded out of her during her commute. At dinner she excused herself to write down plot ideas and new traits for characters. Then she just brought a pad to the table and apologized to Pete before scribbling down several more intriguing thoughts she wanted to ensure she remembered for her novel.

With 10 weeks of vacation time accrued since Pete had started to avoid taking vacations with her, she decided to take several full days off to write. The first day she visited her father, but stopped a dozen times on the two-hour drive to San Diego to make notes for her novel. With that melancholy visit behind her—her father had not even recognized her—she spent several full days writing. The words flowed into sentences, the sentences into paragraphs, the paragraphs into pages, and the pages into chapters. Before she knew it, she had three polished, complete chapters and six more drafted. Even better, through it all she hadn't smoked a single cigarette. She had been jogging less, devoting her time to writing, but she felt great: full of energy, ideas and confidence.

Reading the chapters on the sofa without a pen in hand one warm August night, she tried to read her words with fresh eyes, as a reader would. It was easier to do without a pen in her hand to change a word here or add a comma there. A pen in hand made her feel like an editor, not a reader.

Finishing the third chapter, she set the pages down on her lap. Hesitant to pronounce them good, she had to admit that they were very good. The words sparkled. The ideas came through vividly. The themes and symbols were clear, yet far from obvious. She loved the flawed protagonists, hated yet sympathized with the nuanced villains and was intrigued by the supporting characters. All the characters pulsated with life, complexity and memorable quirks and traits. The story moved forward at a steady, forceful pace that drew the reader along, as if floating down a broad powerful river. It glowed, it sang, it was a pleasure to read. She had trouble believing she had written it.

The key, she realized with a sliver of apprehension, was what agents and editors would think. What she thought amounted to less than nothing. Everyone loved their own writing. Even so, these chapters had to be publishable. If they weren't good, she was no judge of writing. In fact, if they weren't good, she had no judgment at all. They had to be good. If they weren't, she would stop writing because these chapters were as good as she could write.

The next morning she mailed a cover letter, outline of her novel and the three sample chapters to a New York agent, Charles Wood-Byrd. She thought about submitting to her usual 10 agents, but the novel was so good that any agent would have to want to represent it. And, she thought with a rueful smile, if Wood-Byrd rejected it, she could send it to 10 more agents after another round of revisions. Although it was her usual procedure, in this case she could not imagine how she could revise, let alone improve the chapters at all. Every word was perfect.

The rivalry is with yourself.
I try to be better than is possible.
I fight against myself, not against the other.

—Pavarotti

"Toes pointed ahead or slightly toe-in when you break," Adina yelled. "Never toe-out or you're wasting energy."

Dressed in red shorts that brushed his knees and a white Spartans football T-shirt dark with sweat, Pete ran wind sprints at the school's track. The sun cast its first golden rays through the cypresses that lined the eastern side of the practice field, warming the air into the low seventies. It was a pleasant break from the August heat that would come well before noon.

"Push through the ball of the foot, not the toes," Adina called. "Strength comes from the ball of the foot, not the toes! The ball!"

Pete jogged back to the starting line, wondering what he had got himself into.

"Thighs drive vertically. Use your arms more."

Pete nodded at his taskmaster. Toe in, ball of foot, thighs vertical, and arms moving; four brief things, yet so hard to remember, let alone replicate endlessly, sprint after sprint. If he tried to think of it all at once, he'd be lucky to manage two steps before collapsing in a tangled heap. He took a deep breath and crouched again at the starting line as if he was preparing for a play in a game.

Adina set the stopwatch and yelled, "Down! Set! Hike! Hike! Hike!"

Pete drove his legs forward. He pumped his arms bent 90 degrees and moving opposite to his legs as he sprinted down the track. The cool morning air rushed past. His legs pounded off the cinder track in a smooth, recurring motion.

As he jogged back from his latest 40-yard effort, Adina yelled, "Good, good. Four point five seven."

Pete grinned.

"You'll be a touch slower on grass, but you're getting faster." Adina beamed. Her straight, white teeth shone between her thick lips, which, Pete noticed, had a little upturn at either end that made it always appear as if she was about to break into a smile. There was a slight gap between her front teeth, which added a touch of imperfection to her face, yet made it more pleasing to Pete's eyes. "All your hard work is beginning to pay off."

Pete smiled but a sliver of him shied away from the compliment. "You've helped a lot," he said, staring off down the track.

"You're the one who's been working your tail off. Coach says, 'Advice is free, making use of it is the hard part.'"

Pete nodded, uncertain what to say.

"Never thought I'd see the day when a football player worked out with girls," a deep voice yelled.

Pete and Adina spun around to look across the cinder track. A tall, slope-shouldered black teenager stood on the grass verge in gray shorts and a black T-shirt with orange lettering proclaiming, "Heatherdale High, Texas State Champs" across his broad chest: Joe Cain. The muscular arms protruding from the loose shirt were the size of most freshmen's thighs. His shorn head glistened with sweat. Cain's shorts ended just below the knee, revealing calves bulging with muscle. But what caught Pete's eyes the most were Cain's eyes. Set into his dark face, the whites of his eyes glowed like two possessed orbs. The iris of each was smaller than normal, increasing the impact of those bulging white-dominated eyes. The black spot in the center of each was fixed on Pete, like a tiger's on a mouse. Pete was reminded of Mike Singletary, the dominating Hall-of-Fame Chicago Bears' linebacker whose famous predatory eyes led to the network covering NFL games positioning a camera in the end zone just to zoom in on Singletary's otherworldly eyes before each play. Both Singletary and Cain looked like they were going to kill someone—soon.

Sliding his gaze away from those threatening eyes, Pete glanced at Adina, marshaled his courage and demanded, even though he knew the answer, "Who are you?"

"Joe Cain."

Pete had seen Cain working out in June, which Pete had heard was during a short visit Cain and his father had made to meet Coach Paukenan. Now Cain had moved permanently and was preparing for football tryouts, which started Monday.

"Who are you?" Cain challenged.

Pete felt young and weak, but kept such feelings out of his voice as he barked back, "Pete Tomlinson."

"You're one of the boys I'll be replacing."

"Not likely." Pete's voice was flat and cold. He hated Cain already.

Cain smiled, showing perfect white teeth. "Nothing I like better than a challenge, but taking on a linebacker who trains with girls? Doesn't seem hardly fair."

"He's faster than you," Adina yelled, making Pete grin; a grin that vanished the instant she glanced up at him.

"Maybe on a track; never on a football field." Still grinning like a smug leopard, Cain's aggressive, predatory eyes appraised Pete. "You best get your mind around sitting on the bench, Tomlinson because it's either gonna be you or that Jayden Andrews sitting there, not me."

"Keep dreaming. This isn't Texas."

"Nope; Texas has produced more football players than the rest of the country combined."

"And more bullshit."

Enraged, Cain launched himself at Pete.

Never awaken me when you have good news
to announce, because with good news nothing
presses; but when you have bad news, arouse
me immediately, for then there is not an
instant to be lost.

—Napoleon

Julie stumbled home from work exhausted with a headache, dry mouth and a churning stomach. She thought that the later was caused by the catered lunch she'd consumed at Neurosurgery Grand Rounds. She regretted attending. She'd barely heard the talk since she'd been writing down ideas for her novel. If she'd accepted Severn's invitation for lunch with a pharma rep at Cafe La Boheme instead of attending the grand rounds, maybe she wouldn't have the stomach ache.

"Hey, Mom," Pete called from the living room, where he was watching television. "How was your day?"

"Fine, but I'm not feeling the best." Julie flipped through the mail where Pete had dropped it on the kitchen table: bills and junk. "I'm going to crawl off to bed. Can you fend for yourself for dinner? There's brown rice, chicken and stir-fried vegetables left over from last night in the fridge."

"I ate it for a snack when I got home."

"All of it?"

"I'm trying to eat seven small meals a day to add muscle, but no fat. The training info you got me recommended it."

From her food bills, Julie wondered if Pete was eating 70, not seven, meals a day. He turned back to the television, which, Julie noticed, was showing a DVD of a Spartans football game from last year.

"What happened to your arm?" she asked, noticing a long scrape on Pete's left arm, as if he had slid across gravel.

"Guy shoved me."

"Who? Why?"

"Some new kid. No big deal."

Julie decided Pete looked alright and, lacking the energy to pursue the issue, she sighed and turned to head for her bedroom.

"Oh, I almost forgot," Pete called, freezing the DVD between plays, "some guy called from New York."

Julie spun around. "Who was it?"

"I scribbled his name down. Said to call him back Monday; he was leaving for the day."

Julie rushed over to the pad next to the phone in the kitchen and read Pete's scrawl. Charles Wood-Byrd had called; the agent. "Did he say anything?" Julie demanded as she rushed back into the living room.

"Said to call him Monday," Pete repeated, immersed in his analysis of the other team's plays as he watched a pass play again.

Monday? Julie thought with anguish. Two days to wonder whether the agent wanted her novel: two agonizing days. Why had he called on a Friday? Why hadn't Pete asked for more information?

"Pete," she began, ready to rant, but changed her mind even as she began. It wasn't his fault. She stretched her head back and tilted it side to side in an attempt to relax her neck before setting off for her bedroom. Her bed would feel so good.

"Oh," Pete called, "he did say something like, 'he hoped he had what you'd consider to be good news.'"

Betraying her frustration, she yelled, "What does that mean?"

Every minute of the weekend seemed like an hour. At least Julie was on call and it was a busy weekend in the ED for MVAs: motor vehicle accidents. A 35-year-old male had been driving home late Friday night along the 10 and flipped his Mercedes CLK-320 convertible. The car's automatic roll bar deployed and saved his life, escaping with minimal injuries. However, disoriented, he wandered out into traffic and a passing pickup clipped him. He suffered major damage to his lumbar and thoracic spine, left femur, multiple bones in his left hand, and his brain. In a coma, he was cradled in a bed that tilted with a slow but continuous motion from side to side to prevent pressure ulcers—bed sores. He had pulmonary congestion, resulting in labored breathing that sounded as if it was coming from a 90-year-old asthma patient trying to breathe through a straw. He had decerebrate rigidity; his jaws were clenched, his neck retracted and all his limbs extended. His blood pressure was elevated and his pulse slow. Julie performed a craniotomy to remove part of the young man's skull to give his brain room to swell without being crushed. About seven percent of patients in a coma remain unresponsive and Julie feared he would be one of the seven percent.

There was also a three-car collision on the 405 that led to critical injuries. One was in a coma and the other two suffered serious spine damage, although their brains were fine, save for minor concussions. Even so, they would bear careful observation. Nurses would awaken the patients every hour throughout the night to ensure they were lucid and aware as to time, place and identity. If not, it could mean there was bleeding into their brain, which would require immediate surgical intervention. Although most people think neurosurgeons only operate on the brain, they also operate on the spine.

As Julie dictated a report on the last of the MVA casualties she marveled at a society that went ballistic if a single airliner with 350 people crashed or one child was abducted, yet accepted 50,000 people killed on its roads and freeways every year with appalling regularity. Worse, car companies advertised how fast their cars could go, which violated every speed limit in the country, yet no one sued them for encouraging people to break the law.

Julie arrived home late Saturday night and, falling into bed, fell asleep.

As she dreamed, King Carl Gustaf XVI of Sweden in 19th Century formal attire waited for Dr. Julie Stein, medal and diploma for the Nobel Prize in Literature in his left hand. In a low-cut, dark blue gown, Julie rose as the formally attired audience applauded, rising as one to a standing ovation that grew to a crescendo. She slipped out of her row to start down the plush red carpeting of the Stockholm Concert Hall. Beaming and giddy, she knew this was the high point of her life. Even as she reveled in the all-encompassing feeling of accomplishment, the carpeting deepened and her feet grew heavy as she struggled to approach the stage and reach the King with his glittering medal and priceless diploma.

She was getting nowhere. The King with his prizes wasn't any closer. Looking down, she found that her feet had disappeared into the thick red carpet, which held her fast. Worse, she now wore green scrubs and a lab coat, its pockets full of a jangling, unwieldy jumble of prescription pad, pager, cell phone, Blackberry, pens, otoscope, and stethoscope. She struggled to free herself from the ensnaring carpet, but her struggles only ensnared her deeper into the red pile even as her arms were tangled in all the medical paraphernalia in her pockets.

The applause, which had been rolling over her, turned to hisses, boos and screams of derision.

"You quack!"

"Stick to writing prescriptions, not novels!"

"How dare you compare yourself to Chekhov, Maugham or Doyle. You're not even a decent doctor, let alone a writer."

"Hack! Hack! Hack!"

Rising from their velvet-covered seats, the angry crowd closed in.

"Hack! Hack! Hack!"

Julie pushed and kicked to free herself from the carpeting, but to no avail. The crowd's arms pressed in toward her, their fists swinging at her.

"Hack! Hack! Hack!"

She swung a futile fist to defend herself and with a jolt she awoke, shaking, sweating and filled with terror. She was alone in her bed, tangled amidst the blankets and sheets. She had delivered a death blow to her pillow.

"What in the world is that?" Julie asked Pete as he emerged from his room Sunday morning lugging a large orange, nylon bundle.

"A parachute," Pete said as he dropped it on the floor to pull on his sneakers in the front hall.

"No," Julie announced, torn out of her musings on what the agent would say when she called him Monday. "No way, no how, never in my lifetime. In fact, never in your lifetime."

Pete frowned.

"You are not jumping out of an airplane; never."

"I don't plan to, Mom."

"Oh…and you are not jumping off a bridge, building or any other high place. Understood?"

"I'm not jumping off anything. Chill, Mom."

"Then what's it for?" Julie asked, stalking over from the breakfast table to prod the offending nylon chute with her toe. She grimaced as a pain shot through her stomach.

"I wear it to run wind sprints. It helps with my speed for football, and for basketball and baseball, too. I bought it after I read about it in a football-training magazine."

"With what?"

Pete fell silent.

"I told you not to gamble, Pete."

Silence.

"Pete, it's a terrible, dangerous habit."

"It's just a few bucks. Some buddies asked if I wanted to and I figured I'd take a chance. I won."

"That's beside the point. Don't gamble. I've told you that before. Don't you see how dangerous gambling can become? It can ruin your life." Her words had no effect on her son. He waited like a long-experienced commuter resigned to a tardy bus. Julie decided this was not the time to fight the war again over gambling; besides her stomach and head ached. "What does the chute do?"

"It increases resistance and builds muscle faster." He rose, gathered up his chute and, opening the door, said, "I gotta go. Adina's waiting for me."

"Who's Adina?" Julie yelled as Pete jogged out to his car.

"Just a girl."

"What girl? Who is she?"

Pete scrambled into his car and sped away.

There are three difficulties in authorship:
to write anything worth publishing,
to find honest men to publish it, and
to find sensible men to read it.

—Charles Caleb Colton, English cleric and
critic, 1780-1832

Julie awoke at 5 a.m. Monday and wondered how soon she could call Charles Wood-Byrd. Six a.m.? It would be 9 a.m. in New York. But he would know it was 6 a.m. in LA and might think her desperate to call right at the start of the business day. She should wait, maybe even until 7 a.m. LA time so she would appear less eager. That settled it. She would wait until 7 a.m. to call.

With plenty of time, she considered going into work, but knew she wouldn't get any work done until after she'd talked to the agent. With no clinic or early meetings that morning, she rolled over to try to fall back asleep. Cold, she pulled up the comforter. In a few minutes she felt hot, so she shoved the comforter down. The muffled rumble of a truck seeped through the double-glazed windows. Her mind jumped from thought to thought, all to do with writing, agents and publishers, and the future. Cold, she pulled the comforter up. Sleep would not come.

A strong smell of orange came to her, but try as she might, she could not figure out where the odor originated. She hadn't bought oranges in weeks. As she wrinkled her nose to try to rid it of the aroma, which was becoming tiresome, she recalled that several of her clinical trial patients had complained of hallucinations, including olfactory illusions.

Putting the orange smell down to the effect of the trial drugs, she flicked on the light and grabbed a novel off her bedside table, Derek Robinson's *Piece of Cake*. It was one of her father's favorites, a dark comedic take on the life of British Royal Air Force fighter pilots during the Battle of Britain. Her father had recommended it to her years before and her brother, who loved reading military history, recently seconded the recommendation. Engaging, well written and an entertaining combination of drama and black humor, it held Julie's attention for three minutes.

At 5:25, unable to stand it any longer, she got up and tried to take her time showering, brushing her hair and getting dressed. She brushed her teeth three times to try to get rid of the metallic taste in her mouth. It persisted. She knew it was from the drugs she was taking and, if that and the orange smell were the only side effects, she could live with them. Her stomach churned, but she put that down to the time of the month.

As she dallied and delayed, she found that time barely passed. Unfortunately, as a surgeon on call she had long ago learned to get up and out of the house faster than most people took to get out of bed. She swallowed an aspirin for her headache and ate breakfast with slow deliberation, but when she checked the time it wasn't even six yet. She checked her email in her home office and tried to be quiet since Pete was still asleep.

Six o'clock finally, reluctantly came. She shuddered to think of the damage the stress of waiting would do to her body over the painful hour until 7. She could not do it. It would be irresponsible and unhealthy, not to mention impossible. After a superhuman effort, she waited until 6:15 to call Mr. Wood-Byrd. Her hands shook and her heart raced as she paced across the living room carpet, phone in hand.

"Ms. Stein, thanks for calling," a smooth, cultured tenor answered after an efficient sounding English—or was the accent Canadian?—secretary had put Julie through. "How are you?"

"I'm well," Julie said, eager to get past the pleasantries.

"Thank you for returning my call."

"It was no problem."

"Now, let me find your file. Ah, just a moment, my desk is a bit of a no-man's land at the moment. The copy for all the fall publishers' catalogues are due next week and I have to review the text for all of my authors. Bit of a chore, but one must make certain every word is shipshape and correct."

Julie writhed in an agony of suspense. Her stomach churned and her head ached.

"Ah, yes, here it is. Well, the long and short of it is, I received your novel and, the truth be told, rather loved it."

Julie stopped pacing. The world stopped. Someone liked her writing. Not just someone, an agent, a New York agent. And not just liked, loved. Her entire life telescoped down to this point; this wonderful, exhilarating, splendid moment.

"I must reluctantly and ruefully admit to one minor problem," Mr. Wood-Byrd's voice cut into Julie's glorious trance like an ax.

Julie stood transfixed. What could be wrong? Possible problems stampeded through her mind unbidden. He loved the chapters she had sent but he thought there was no market for that sort of novel? The memory of Theodore Geisel, better known as Dr. Seuss, sprang into her mind. He had submitted his work to publishers who had told him they loved his work but that it would never sell, at least until one editor brought a manuscript home and his children wouldn't give it back. Or maybe the market was far too difficult for new authors and Wood-Byrd was only accepting novelists who had previously published. The endless possibilities that would destroy her writing career before it started coursed through her mind leaving their dark, gloomy trails behind.

"I fear I was rather indiscreet with your chapters," Wood-Byrd said. "May I enquire whether you have availed yourself of the opportunity to submit it to any other agents of literary works?"

Julie felt a rush of relief. Whatever the problem was, she could honestly say, "No."

"Any houses?"

"Houses?"

"Publishing houses?"

"No."

"I am greatly relieved to hear that particular piece of information."

"What's wrong?" Julie asked, unable to stand the suspense any longer. She felt dizzy, faint and a rising nausea.

"I am rather embarrassed."

Julie paced, fighting the urge to scream at him to just tell her what had happened.

"I was reading your chapters and an old friend of mine from my Choate days came in to lunch with me," Wood-Byrd said. "He asked what I was reading, since I was reluctant to stop, and when I told him, he asked to look it over. Without thinking, I handed him what I had read; mainly so I could finish reading the chapter in which I was immersed. I am afraid we both read your sample chapters and outline in their entirety. We never did make it to lunch. Missed a rather good leg of lamb at Café Boulud; comes with splendid *pomme frites.*"

When he didn't continue, Julie said, "That sounds good." What was the problem?

"Yes, I've had the lamb before…"

"No, I meant I thought it was good that you liked my chapters."

"I pray you will think it is good."

"I'm sure I will," Julie said, far from sure of anything.

"You see, my old Choate friend is Jonathan Sharpe, the founder, CEO and publisher of Kira House Press."

Julie stared out the living room window from where she stood rooted to the carpet. She couldn't believe her ears.

"He made an offer to buy the book on the spot with a more than reasonable advance," Wood-Byrd reported, "but I was forced to my great embarrassment to confess to him that I did not yet have the honor of representing the author."

"But you do, you can," Julie rushed to say. "If you want to, I mean."

"Oh, I am extremely relieved to hear you say that. It was rather embarrassing all around. I had a rather sleepless weekend wondering how you would respond to my amateurish indiscretion and spot of news. I was hoping you would call at 9 am. The past quarter hour has been rather an infernal interlude."

A competitor will find a way to win.
Competitors take bad breaks and use them to
drive themselves just that much harder.
Quitters take bad breaks and use them as
reasons to give up. It's all a matter of pride.

—Nancy Lopez, professional golfer, b. 1957

Pete's eyes flicked over to Jayden on his left and then to Joe Cain on his right. An eye-searing August sun glared down on the final day of tryouts for the Santa Maria High School football team. Most of the walk-ons had been cut and the team had taken shape around a core of the previous year's juniors, now seasoned seniors. The sinewy sophomore, Manny Ortiz made backup safety. He'd at least get to play a few downs this year. A couple of positions were still in doubt, including the linebackers. Coach Paukenan's defensive scheme used two linebackers and he had three talented players for the position: Pete, Jayden Andrews and the transfer from Texas, Joe Cain.

The trio stood at the end zone ready to sprint 40 yards in front of the coaches with their stopwatches. The coaches would time them at 10-, 20- and 40-yard intervals to measure their explosion off the line and the time to their top speed. All three players wore grey T-shirts dark with sweat from their second practice of the day, which almost hid the words "Spartans Football" in dark green on their chests.

"Down!" the defensive coach barked.

The linebackers crouched as if they were on the field during a game, ready to launch themselves down the field at an opposing running back.

"Set! Hike! Hike!"

All three players burst across the goal line and raced down the field. As Adina had taught him, Pete focused on keeping his legs driving, his arms correctly positioned and his body at the perfect angle for speed. His vision narrowed to the strip of turf before him.

Before he knew it, 40 yards flew by. He slowed and turned to trot back to Coach Paukenan, who held a stopwatch at the 40-yard line.

"Good, good work, Tomlinson!" Paukenan yelled. "4.50. Excellent speed! Jayden and Cain, both 4.55. Excellent work, excellent!"

Pete grinned, relieved that his training had paid off. He grabbed a towel from a metal bench to wipe the sweat off his face, avoiding the persistent acne near his nose. Even Amanda's ministrations failed to control the acne anymore.

Coach Paukenan strode off to consult his defensive coach. Behind them, players hit tackling dummies, hit blocking sleds and did the mirror drill with another coach.

"You and me, Tomlinson," Jayden whispered to Pete as they drank from water bottles that had been brought out to them by a couple of freshmen water girls. Cain chugged water a few steps away as they awaited their coach's decision. Cain smiled confidently when Pete glanced at him.

Pete looked over at the concrete bleachers where a spattering of girlfriends, parents, friends, and boosters sat watching. Amanda perused a magazine. Several rows above her, Adina wore a simple white dress, setting her apart from the other students, all of whom wore T-shirts and shorts.

"Gentlemen, over here," Coach Paukenan called. The three linebackers trotted over to him. "You made this decision a tough one. You'd all make it on the first squad at any other high school in the state, but I'm lucky—or unlucky—enough to have to choose two as starters. The odd man out will have to beat out one of our tackles for one of their spots."

Pete stood, hands on hips, waiting. He did not want to be a tackle. His face was impassive, but his stomach and mind churned with hopes and fears that would be settled in the next few few seconds.

"I'd like to play all three of you, but I don't want to change our defensive scheme that worked so well for us last year," Coach said, looking from Jayden to Pete to Cain. "Before I announce my decision, I want to make it perfectly clear that my decision is only for this week. Every week I'll be watching all three of you at practice and I'll play the best two for that week. So don't think whoever I pick are the starting linebackers for anything more than the first game. Understood?"

"Understood," all three linebackers barked back.

Pete wished coach would just tell them his decision.

"I also want it understood that it was a difficult decision."

Coach looked at each of them in turn again. Pete wanted to yell at him to damn well tell them his decision, but swallowed hard to stifle the urge.

"I'll rotate all three of you as our tight ends, as needed, so even if you aren't a linebacker, you'll still play."

Pete knew tight end was a consolation prize; no way he wanted it. He turned his full attention on Coach Paukenan. Who would it be? All his hard work, and the steroids, had to have made a difference. If not, what was the point of either?

The price of greatness is responsibility.

—Winston Churchill

As Julie squeezed the handle on the cutting forceps to break through the sphenoid bone, she felt and heard the instrument snap.

"Broken," she announced as she withdrew the eight-inch instrument from the patient's nostril. She handed it to the attending resident. "Make sure nothing broke off in her."

The resident took the forceps and laid them on a tray draped with a blue, sterile towel. As the resident checked the broken instrument, a blue-gowned OR nurse handed Julie another long-handled set of tiny cutting scissors, angled to fit through the nasal cavity.

Watching on the video screen across from her, which showed the image of the inside of the patient's sphenoid sinus cavity via a tube-like endoscope, Julie threaded the new instrument into position against the bone that separated the cavity from the tumor she was seeking to remove from the base of the patient's brain.

Julie squeezed, felt the instrument give and announced, "This one broke, too. She definitely doesn't have osteoporosis."

The resident and nurses in the white-tiled operating room laughed.

"Let's try breaking through the old fashioned way," Julie decided, pointing at a bone punch; a chisel-like instrument that lay on the tray beside the OR nurse.

Julie looked up at the white-faced clock on the wall, which had been started the moment the mother of three had been put under. The longer a patient was under, the greater the risk of something going wrong. "Call the patient's husband and tell him everything's going fine. It's just taking a little longer than expected. Tell him she's doing great."

"Should I tell him she doesn't have osteoporosis?" the nurse asked, her smile hidden behind her surgical mask.

"I think we can leave that part out," Julie said with a chuckle. She winced as a cramp struck her stomach.

The nurse called the waiting area.

"All here," the resident announced, straightening up after his forceps inspection.

"Want to give this a try?" Julie asked the resident, trying to ignore the crescendo of pain in her stomach.

"Sure."

Julie handed him the bone punch, shifting to the side to allow the resident in closer. Keeping intent eyes on him, she watched him begin to work. Even as she watched, the urge to use the toilet mounted. She had eaten her usual bagel with cream cheese breakfast, but even as she tried to ignore the urge, she realized she would have to leave, now, right now.

"Can you get through the bone to the tumor?" she asked the resident. She winced at the pain in her stomach, buckling at the waist as if she'd been punched.

"Sure."

"I have to step out for a minute. If you run into any trouble, stop and wait for me. Understood? Any trouble at all, stop."

Before the bewildered resident even answered, Julie rushed from the OR suite, across the hall past the washing station and into the physicians' locker-room. She just made it to the toilet.

Sitting at her desk before clinic late that morning, Julie took another anti-diarrheal and wondered what she could have eaten to cause such a problem. Nothing came to mind. Hoping it was not something she and Pete had eaten, she called him on his cell. He was fine.

Her mouth parched, she drank yet another glass of water to alleviate the dry mouth and maintain her hydration from the diarrhea. Her head pounded. Her stomach ached as if someone with a sharp rake was enthusiastically gardening in it. She asked Sandy to either reschedule her clinic patients or find another neurosurgeon to cover for her, so she could go home and die in peace.

"I hope you feel better," Sandy said.

"I can cover for you," Rick Severn offered as he ambled down the corridor, having overheard their conversation. "You alright?"

"Just a touch of food poisoning," Julie said, eager to head home.

"If you came out for lunch with me, this would never happen," Severn said, wagging an admonishing finger at her. "Need a ride home?"

"No thanks. If you can just see my patients in clinic this afternoon, I'd be in your debt."

"Debt enough to come to lunch with me?"

"With you, yes; with drug reps, no."

"You look like hell," Alan McGhee said as he hobbled up Julie's driveway, Macduff straining on the end of his leather leash.

"Nice to see you, too," Julie said, managing a grin as she slammed her car door. She winced and bent at the waist as another spasm ripped through her stomach.

Macduff roared, but Alan shushed him with a snap of the leash, which earned Alan a glare from his short companion.

"Can I help you inside?" Alan asked. "What's wrong?"

"Run-of-the-mill food poisoning. I'll be fine."

Her hands shook as he helped her up the steps. She dropped her keys as another spasm engulfed her stomach. Alan picked them up and opened the front door, helping her into the living room and onto the sofa.

"Can I get you something for your stomach?" he asked.

"Can you look in the bathroom medicine cabinet and see if we have anything?"

Alan returned holding a plastic medicine cup full of pink liquid. "Bottoms up."

Julie drank the concoction and regretted not having something stronger for stomach trouble in the house.

"I couldn't help noticing," Alan began, then changed course, "I'm an Army officer so I tend to be a little blunt, but...you have a lot of drugs in your medicine cabinet."

Julie cradled her stomach, keeping her hands on it, which soothed it somewhat. "I *am* a doctor. How's your knee?"

"Fine, fine." Alan shifted on the sofa. "When will Pete be home?"

Julie looked at her watch. "Not for a while, but I'll be fine. I don't want to keep you."

"You aren't. I was just exercising my knee, and Macduff." He sat silent, not moving. Then, as if he had decided something, he turned to her and asked, "Are you sick? I mean, not just stomach trouble, you have a medicine cabinet full of prescriptions and...."

Julie wished he hadn't seen the pill bottles.

When she didn't reply, he rushed on, "I know it's none of my business, but I couldn't help noticing the names on the bottles. Twenty-ten vision and all, and I've commanded a lot of young men, and some of them have gotten into trouble with drugs, and..."

"I'm not in trouble with any drugs," Julie said, interrupting his string of nervous thoughts. There was no easy way to explain. "I better get some rest. Thanks for your help."

Everything I've ever done
was out of fear of being mediocre.

—Chet Atkins, US guitarist and Country
Music Hall of Fame inductee, 1924-2001

September

Sitting in the bleachers at Pete's first game of the season, Julie felt far from well. Even though she had already drunk a bottle of water, her mouth felt so dry the rugae on the roof of her mouth felt like corrugated metal. Worse, her teeth felt as if they were made of aluminum. She had thought she'd get used to the metallic taste; she'd been wrong. The odd sensation had made her less inclined to eat, since everything took on a distressing metallic aftertaste. Not that she felt like eating anyway. Her stomach had been upset, only kept in check by regular doses of anti-diarrhea medication, which dehydrated her and compounded the constant headache that lurked to varying painful degrees throughout her head like a roving pain monster.

Even though her health had not been good, she and Pete had enjoyed a pleasant Rosh Hashanah dinner with her mom and her brother's and sister's families in Carlsbad, where her older sister lived. Julie had not eaten much, nibbling on some challah bread. At the Sabbath services, she had managed to make it through the long service without having to go to the bathroom, much to her surprise. To try not to think of her stomach during the service, she had considered whether she should find some moving water on which to sprinkle breadcrumbs, which were supposed to represent her sins being washed away. As she considered the issue, she was far from certain whether taking the drugs from her clinical trial was a sin. How could it be when it led to such exquisite prose?

Watching Pete's game, she craved a cigarette. Smoking was not allowed in the stands; not that she should be smoking anywhere. She had not jogged in a week. She should be training for the LA Marathon, but she felt far from able to jog a mile, let alone 26. At least she still had plenty of time before the marathon in March.

As she half watched the game—the Spartans' offense was on the field and Pete had just made a diving catch as tight end, so he probably wouldn't be involved in the next play—she chastised herself for how she had handled or, more accurately, mishandled, Alan's discovery of her cache of trial drugs in her medicine cabinet. She had been far from well when he had made his discovery. Even so, she could have behaved better. She did not want Alan to think she was shutting him out, but she felt far from comfortable talking about her drug taking, let alone about her dream of becoming a novelist. She knew from past experience that telling someone you wanted to be a novelist brought indulgent smiles, as if you were five years old and had just proclaimed your intention to be a prima ballerina for the Bolshoi.

At least her writing was progressing well. By taking the drug cocktail, she was able to write and write well. She hated to get her hopes up, but she had completed two more chapters of her novel and, taking as objective a stance as possible, she believed they were good, maybe even great. She had never written anything as good and much of what she had read published today paled in comparison. Wood-Byrd and the publisher would have to love them.

It was the fourth quarter and Pete had made three individual tackles, as well as two receptions at tight end. She had learned a great deal about football during the past 12 years since he had first donned helmet, shoulder pads and size eight cleats as a Tiny-Mite in the local Pop Warner football program as a 38-pound, four year old, and she knew he was playing well.

She could see Tom Tomlinson, her tall, muscular ex-husband and his new busty wife, Christy, six rows down from her and to the right a few seats. Every time Pete made a play, Tom and Christy rose to cheer. Julie was happy that Tom had made the game, but she felt that a part of her maternal rights were being usurped every time Christy cheered. Who did she think she was, his mother?

Julie's stomach rumbled. She had taken some medication after dinner to make certain she could make it through the game, but she realized that she should have doubled the dosage. Even as she dug in her bag for more pills, the defense with Pete at middle linebacker trotted onto the field for the final plays of the fourth quarter.

Julie winced. Her stomach ached. Then it hurt. Watching as the teams lined up, she looked up at the clock; 2:06 left in the game. Score: Pete's Spartans 21, Sutherland Sabres 20, thanks to a blocked point-after.

Julie willed her stomach to cooperate. She had to see the end of the game. Pete might make a play. She had to stay two more minutes.

The Sabres ran a play, but Julie couldn't follow it.

She told herself that she could make it. She had to. Pete was on the field.

Pain stabbed through her belly.

Just one minute. She had to stay.

More pain. Sweat bathed her body. She suppressed a groan, wincing from the agony in her gut. Why did the last two minutes of a game take so long to play?

Giving in, she rose and, excusing herself past irritated parents and fans trying to watch the final moments of the game, she rushed out of her aisle and up the metal stairs with clanging footfalls in a desperate charge to the bathroom.

The Sabres were on the Spartans' 12-yard line, threatening. Pete read the signal from Coach Paukenan; single linebacker blitz.

Pete returned to the defensive huddle and ordered, "Orange 93; Orange 93."

The huddle broke. Pete took his position in the middle of the backfield. Jayden was to his left on the open side of the field, just past the left end. Pete glimpsed Cain pacing the sideline, shaking his hands and jumping up and down as he eagerly awaited action. Not in my lifetime, Pete thought. Having won a starting position there was no way he was going to lose it—ever.

Pete glanced up at the clock: 36 seconds.

The Sabre quarterback started his count.

Pete lined up on the balls of his feet, crouched and ready, elbows tucked in as Adina had taught him.

"Down! Set!"

Pete kept his eyes focused on the quarterback, anger and hatred rising in him. As the single linebacker blitzing, he had to get to the quarterback. The game depended on it.

Pete moved in to line up with the slot between the Sabre tackle and left end. With two wide receivers on Jayden's side of the field and one on the Spartans' right, Pete guessed the play would go to his left. He hoped to catch the quarterback looking to his right to throw while Pete charged in from his blindside.

"Hike!"

The center snapped the ball. The quarterback took the snap. Pete slipped through the narrow gap between two of his own lineman. The quarterback took a step back with the ball. Pete turned his shoulders and shoved his way between the Sabre tackle and end. In an instant he was through. His eyes locked on the quarterback, who looked right— away from Pete—at his two receivers sprinting down field. Pete grinned; the quarterback hadn't yet learned to look first where he wasn't going to throw. Before the thought left his mind, Pete had covered the two yards between him and his quarry.

Pete blindsided the unsuspecting quarterback. He hit him around the waist, at the same time slamming his right arm down into the quarterback's throwing arm and hammering the Sabre to the turf. As Pete rolled over, he saw the ball bouncing away across the turf: a sack and a fumble.

A roar went up from the hometown crowd. Jayden dove on the loose ball to smother it and claim it—and a last-second win—for the Spartans.

"Great play, Pete," Tom Tomlinson told his son. Pete had just emerged from the locker room in jeans and a gray T-shirt after the coach's post-game talk and a shower.

Pete's dad was dressed in Spartans dark green and white like most of the fans. "You've become a better player than I ever was." He threw a muscular arm around Pete and added, "That working out has really paid off. You're in the best shape I've ever seen you."

Pete beamed under the paternal praise. He *had* been working hard.

"You're even catching the ball better," Pete's father told him. "And you're turning up field faster after each reception."

"Great game, Pete," Christy said. Petite, with short blond hair and a figure that was the result of an addiction to aerobics, tennis and swimming, Christy reminded Pete of an airheaded cheerleader. Outgoing and bubbly, she'd even be the life of a funeral. Even so, he found it hard not to like her, especially since she made his dad happy.

"Have you seen Mom?" Pete asked, trying to look over, around or through the crowd of parents, students and players in the wide hall outside the locker room, which had the Spartans' emblem emblazoned on its green door. A table just down the hall manned by students sold Spartans baseball caps, jerseys, T-shirts, buttons, pom-poms, sweatshirts, hoodies, cups, and all manner of Spartans paraphernalia.

"Julie was sitting behind us," Christy said, rising onto her toes to survey the crowd.

"I haven't seen her since near the end of the game," Pete's dad said, looming over his petite wife. An ex-tackle who had made it for a year in the pros, Tom still kept in shape with a steady regimen of jogging, swimming and biking that kept him looking far younger than his 46 years.

Pete's mom appeared down the hall, hurrying toward them through the crowd.

"Sorry," she said. "I ran into some people I know and couldn't get away."

Pete looked as his mother, waiting for her to say something.

"Ready to go?" she asked Pete.

Pete's hopes collapsed. Hadn't she seen the game? The last play? The sack and the fumble recovery? He won the game. His mom had already turned to say hello to his dad and Christy.

"Great game, Pete," the safety Manny called as he rushed past hand-in-hand with a freshman cheerleader.

"Enjoy the game?" Pete's dad asked his mom.

"Very much," Julie said, smiling up at her son. "We should get going, though. It's getting late and you must be tired."

Pete nodded, hiding his disappointment. What could a mom know about football?

As she lay in bed that night, Julie was forced to the conclusion that it was the side effects of the drug cocktail that were causing her problems. She might have a bug, the flu or some other horrid little bacteria or virus, but her symptoms didn't fit the presentation for any condition of which she'd heard. Worse, her headache, stomach trouble, olfactory hallucinations, and metallic mouth matched the side effects of the trial's drug regimen. She had taken her blood pressure when she arrived home and found it elevated; another side effect of the trial drugs. She would have to take diuretics to keep the hypertension under control, even if they would dehydrate her even more on top of what the diarrhea was already doing to her body. The olfactory hallucinations were becoming more common as she smelled oranges, fish and, during one unpleasant episode, manure when nothing to produce such odors was present. There was nothing she could do about them, but such smells were a small price to pay to write like Shakespeare. She considered the risk of a TIA or stroke, but her patients had been on the drugs for six months before any of them suffered either, and they were far older, weaker and sicker than she was. Far from certain that the first patient's stroke or the second patient's TIA had even been caused by the trial's drugs, she thought that the odds of such events for her were insignificant.

Even so, as she rolled over in an attempt to make her stomach more comfortable, she tried to determine why the side effects from the trial drugs were affecting her more than they appeared to have affected the trial's subjects. The patients in the trial had complained of the same symptoms, but none had appeared to be serious until the stroke and TIA. None of the patients had asked to be taken off the trial and she had needed to prescribe minimal drugs to counteract their headaches, diarrhea, hypertension, and liver problems.

She knew that the same drug could affect people differently. The same dosage of a drug given to two patients could cure the disease in one patient while the other patient experienced debilitating side effects and no curative effect. As research into genetics and proteinomics—the study of how genes express proteins—advanced, it was becoming clearer that disease was as individual as fingerprints. Every case of cancer, asthma, heart disease or Alzheimer's was different, and every patient responded differently to treatment. In the future, Julie was certain, treatments would be individualized for each patient.

Julie also knew that some patients were far from thorough, let alone consistent in communicating what was happening to them when they were undergoing treatment. Some patients complained about every little side effect while others were stoic beyond her comprehension.

She flipped the pillow over to seek a more comfortable resting place for her throbbing head. There was another answer; if she had been facing the terror and identity-robbing symptoms of Alzheimer's, she would have been more than willing to put up with far worse than a dry mouth, headaches, diarrhea and hallucinations for a chance to regain even the semblance of a normal life. If she wanted to publish a novel, she would just have to put up with the same nagging side effects as her trial subjects had endured. She hoped to finish her novel soon. Then she could come off the drugs before the side effects worsened, let alone before the risk of a stroke increased to any appreciable degree.

The party Saturday night was at the home of the Spartans' quarterback, whose parents had driven out to Rancho Mirage for the weekend, trusting in their 23-year-old son to chaperone their 18-year-old son's party. Little chaperoning was being done. The 23 year old was far more interested in a well-developed 18-year-old, 112-pound senior cheerleader who had drunk a little more than the legal limit—for a 300-pound lineman—than in doing any chaperoning.

Pete had drunk a carefully considered beer in violation of his strict diet, not to mention in violation of the law and his mom's rules. He felt he deserved it, not to mention his teammate's intense pressure to toast his game-winning sack and forced fumble. Surrounded by roaring teammates and students, including Amanda, he drained his lager.

The enormous Johnson, their star tackle and the baseball team's stalwart catcher, was leading and winning a beer-drinking contest in one corner of the living room. Pete had been invited, even razzed into participating, but he stood his ground, as usual. Years before he would have drunk a case of beer, but now, his sights on college and the pros, he reigned in his natural impulsiveness and focused on the long-term. It was hard, but it would be worth it.

Looking out the back window at the lit backyard, Pete saw that several players had enticed three drunken girls into skinny dipping in the pool. Sanchez, the tackle, was passed out in a pool chair. Someone had put a black bra over his head like Mickey Mouse ears.

The music engulfing his ears, Pete strolled into the kitchen and scanned the chips, pretzels and cold pizza on the granite-topped island. He was considering which team to put $100 on for the weekend's football games in an attempt to make up for a loss the weekend before, when a voice shouted in his ear through the music, "Great play, Pete."

He turned and looked into a pair of dark eyes. Out of her usual shorts and track singlet, Adina wore a tight white sweater and faded blue jeans that accented her long, shapely legs.

"Thanks," Pete said, glancing over Adina's shoulder to where he could see Amanda talking with Danny Doyle in the living room near the fireplace. It was more than 80 degrees in the house. Even so, someone had lit the logs in the fireplace. Danny leaned in close to Amanda, his mouth an inch from her right ear and his right arm draped across her shoulder. Neither of them noticed the sparks the fire spit out at regular intervals, bouncing off their pant legs before dying on the hearthrug.

"How's the track team doing?" Pete yelled, leaning toward Adina to be heard above Linkin' Park's "Breaking the Habit," which boomed out from tiny white speakers attached to the walls in the student-packed living room.

"Should make State again this year," Adina shouted back. She leaned in toward Pete so he could feel the heat of her body against his. Her eyes narrowed and she asked, "Loud."

He nodded.

"Hot."

He nodded.

"Want to go out on the deck?"

He nodded. He followed her out, marveling at how her hips swung from side to side as if they were on the smoothest pistons ever designed. She looked as if she had been created with curves and no straight lines—and what wonderful curves they were.

Having given up on sleep because of her sore stomach, Julie sat in her bed, laptop on a pillow perched on her thighs, writing late into the night. The words came easily and well. It was as if she had been born to write this novel. It was all so natural and easy; as if the characters had taken over her story and were writing the novel themselves, dictating it to her through her fingers. The house was quiet as she tapped away, adding scene after scene.

Sipping Orange Pekoe with a dash of sugar in it from the American Association of Neurological Surgeons mug on her walnut bedside table, she reread the paragraph she'd just written. After a few words, the belief that she had written the words left her. The writing was too good. How could she have written such perfect words?

Mug down. Fingers to keyboard. Start next scene. This is Heaven.

There are no gains without pains.

—Benjamin Franklin

"You didn't tell me this crap would make me lose my hair," Pete roared at Mike as the science geek arrived before school to drop off Pete's latest supply of steroids.

"You never asked me about side effects," Mike countered as he stood on the front steps of Pete's house. Pete's mom was already at work.

"I look like a fucking monk," Pete raged. Anger coursed through him and he felt his arms tightening with the pleasing thought of pummeling Mike into a black, blue and red lump of broken bones and battered flesh. Pete reached up to feel the bald spot forming on the back of his head. He had noticed it when he returned from a run the day before to discover that his head was burning: the sun had burned his scalp. As he felt the bald spot, his anger reached new heights.

"Easy, Pete, I've got the solution to that little problem, and the acne, too."

"Amanda gave me stuff for the acne; hasn't done a damn bit of good."

Unfazed, Mike set his black backpack down on the top step and dug around in it. He extracted a plastic bottle and two tubes. "Put this on the bald spot twice a day and your worries are over. For the acne, try these; problem solved."

"What are they?"

"Just what you need."

"What are they?" Pete yelled, stepping toward Mike, who backed against the side of the house.

"Settle down. Truth be told, Rogaine and some prescription acne treatment."

"Rogaine?"

"You can buy it yourself or have me do the embarrassing part."

Pete considered, his rage simmering. "You made me lose my hair; you buy it." Pete eyed the clear-skinned Mike. "How'd you get a prescription for acne?"

"Friend of mine had acne; his doctor gave him a prescription for it. I changed the refill number from 2 to 20; simple."

"What happens when it runs out?"

Mike smiled as if explaining something to a child. "Lot of my friends have acne."

Julie waited for her prescriptions, perusing novels in the drugstore's book section. She needed more powerful drugs to counteract the side effects of the drug regimen. She had to hold her body together until she finished her novel: just until then.

She skimmed the plots paraphrased on the back of a few novels and snorted in disgust at their similarity. Several of the mysteries were not who-dun-its, in which the reader was given clues to try to figure out who the murderer was, à la Agatha Christie. From the blurbs on the back, most were stories of psychotic killers with little apparent motive who ended up closing in on the detective/private investigator/coroner/psychologist/hero/heroine intent on killing them. The hero then had to save themselves by killing the killer. The psychotic killer and the hero became the same; murderers. The romances also all were cut from the same boilerplate: a headstrong, accomplished woman coming out of a bad relationship meets a man who is handsome but has some drawback—just lost his wife, has a son/daughter who takes all his time, is busy with a booming business, or has just emerged damaged from his own bad relation-ship—which is remedied just in time to "heal" the woman of all her past pain. Even without drugs, her writing had to be better than most of this drivel.

"Hello, Julie," a beaming Alan McGhee called as he ambled along the aisle toward her.

She smiled and said hello. They asked after each other's ailments: his knee, her dog-bitten foot, and her stomach. All were healed or healing.

"Stein, pharmacy pick-up for Stein," came the announcement over the PA system.

"More prescriptions?" Alan asked, levity in his voice but not, Julie noticed, in his eyes.

"Yes," Julie replied, regretting he'd spotted her.

"Are you alright?"

"Fine." Couldn't he just mind his own business?

He looked concerned and a touch confused. She wasn't handling this well.

He said, "I was just worried."

"No need to be."

Alan looked into her eyes, waiting for an explanation. How could she explain?

She put on her best smile and said, "Female problems, you know?"

Football is, after all, a wonderful way
to get rid of your aggressions
without going to jail for it.

—Heywood Hale Broun, US sportswriter,
1918-2001

Pete sprinted along the defensive line tracking the running back opposite him. Pete's eyes were locked on the back across the jumble of linemen locked in clumsy, brutal embraces in the Trenches. Accelerating, Pete burst from around the end of the line and angled downfield. The running back, cradling the ball in his left arm, sprinted in an arc as he tried to get around Pete before being tackled or forced out of bounds.

The running back was fast, but Pete had the angle. Before the back had made it two yards downfield, Pete forced him out of bounds. Even as the ball-carrier pulled up, Pete slammed into the back, sending him tumbling down hard onto the turf. He came to an abrupt, jarring stop under a metal bench.

Pete halted, glaring down at the other player and yelled, "Get up! Come on! Get up!"

Furious, the back scrambled out from under the bench. As he rose, he hurled the ball at Pete. The football bounced off Pete's chest, ending up a dozen feet away.

"What the hell you doing?!" the back yelled, his facemask clicking and jarring against Pete's facemask.

Pete pushed the back hard with both of his taped hands. This time the back was ready. He shoved Pete back, hard.

"Break it up!" boomed the commanding voice of Coach Paukenan.

Pete shoved the back again. He was setting his feet to launch himself yet again at the other player when a strong arm wrapped around his chest.

"Break it up!" Paukenan ordered. "It's a route drill, Tomlinson. No hitting."

Full of rage, Pete strained against the coach's arm.

"Calm down!"

Pete pushed against the coach's arm, glaring at the back.

"He's on your team. I don't want anyone hurt today."

Pete's entire focus was on the back; on hurting him, bad.

"You're done for the day, Tomlinson. Hit the showers. Now! Right now!"

"It wasn't even a game," Coach Paukenan explained to Julie on the sidelines while assistant coaches continued the practice at Santa Maria High. "He ran a back out of bounds and clocked him a good five yards off the field. No reason. I'm all for aggressiveness, but that was way beyond what's legal, let alone in a drill to practice routes. He's done for today."

Knowing Pete would want to know, Julie asked, "And tomorrow?"

"He can come back tomorrow, but he better keep his temper under control," Paukenan warned. "I'll be keeping a close eye on him."

"Is the other boy alright?"

"Bruised, but fine. Could have been worse. He wasn't wearing a full set of pads and wasn't expecting it. Ended up under a bench or your son might have killed him. I had to break it up."

Julie nodded.

The coach returned to his other charges as Julie walked over and looked down at a sullen Pete who slumped on a bench. He had changed into shorts and his Bears jersey, but his hair was still wet with sweat or had he bothered to shower?

"What happened?"

Pete sighed. "I just hit a guy," he said without even a hint of remorse.

"Out of bounds."

"I misjudged where the sideline was. Let's go."

He rose, head and shoulders above Julie.

"Coach said it wasn't a hitting play."

"I forgot. It's just instinct. I hit people. It's no big deal."

"It didn't sound like 'no big deal' to Coach Paukenan."

Pete and Julie drove home together since Pete's car was in the garage after not starting that morning. They drove the short distance in silence. Once home, Pete retreated to his room to brood.

At dinner Julie raised the issue again.

"I won't do it again, alright?" Pete said, anger in his voice.

"Alright, but I'd like to know why you did it this time."

"It was just a late hit. It's happened before."

"Coach doesn't kick you out of practice for just a late hit."

Pete fell silent as he dug into his spaghetti. Julie took a bite of garlic bread. It tasted dry and metallic. Her taste buds turned everything metallic, but with the new drugs she was taking for her stomach at least she was able to eat, as long as she ignored the illusionary smell of fish that assailed her nostrils.

She wondered if Pete's behavior had anything to do with the letters from college coaches and athletic directors he continued to receive; "We have heard from many sources that you are an outstanding prospect as a student-athlete at a major college," "Our entire coaching staff has been assembling a list of the top high school players in the country. Pete, you are one of those players," and "Your junior year at Santa Maria was exceptional and I'm certain your senior year will be even better. Many high school players dream about being in your position." How couldn't that inflate Pete's ego? Why shouldn't he hit as hard as he could, play as hard as he could and devote himself entirely to football?

"Coach said they had to pull you off the other boy," Julie said, hoping at least to find out what had happened. Then she could decide what to do about it. "Did the other boy say or do something to you?"

"I just got carried away. It won't happen again."

Julie was not going to get to the bottom of this, she realized, especially not tonight. "I hope not or we'll have to reconsider you playing football."

Pete's eyes flicked up to glare at her. His hand on his fork clenched, showing white knuckles. His face, usually so open and friendly, turned hard and reddened, accenting the acne around his nose and across his forehead. "I'm playing football."

Julie met his cold stare. "If you get into any more trouble you're not."

"No fucking way I'm not playing!" Pete screamed, jumping to his feet red-faced and full of rage.

"Never, ever swear at me, Peter Moshe Tomlinson."

"You don't decide whether I play football," Pete stormed.

"I'm your mother. I do decide. You can still play baseball and basketball."

"I'm playing football!"

"That's enough, Pete."

Pete shoved the table, rattling the dishes and upsetting his glass of water. He spun on his heal and stalked off down the hall to his room. The door slammed as Julie sat at the kitchen table, stunned as water cascaded off the table from Pete's overturned glass onto the tile floor.

"It's just football," Tom said when Julie called her ex-husband later that night. "It's a tough, brutal game. You get fired up and want to kill whoever you're playing against."

"It was a practice," Julie said, her exasperation at his attitude showing. "It was his own teammate for Heaven's sake."

"Doesn't matter. You always want to do your best. You want to win, beat the other guy, show you're the best. I made my fair share of out-of-bounds hits."

"In practice?"

"Especially in practice; trying to impress the coach with my aggressiveness so I could start the next game."

Julie paused to take this in. She was forced to admit that Tom knew far more about this area of her son's life than she did, even after she'd spent thousands of hours over the past decade watching

Pete at practices and in games. For some reason, the mentality of the sport, the brutality and quest to win at all costs still eluded her.

Tom laughed and said, "Dick Butkus, the Bear's Hall of Fame linebacker once said, 'I'm not so mean. I wouldn't ever go out to hurt anybody deliberately—unless it was, you know, important, like a league game or something.'"

"Pete's being mean in practice," Julie countered. "And…"

"And what?"

Julie debated whether to tell Tom. "He gets upset at me over nothing."

"Is this a sudden change?"

"Over the past few weeks."

"He's not taking steroids is he?"

"Of course not."

"Sounds like it might be 'roid rage."

"Pete? That's crazy. The district has strict drug testing. I have to sign a form every year so Pete can play, which includes allowing him to be randomly tested."

Tom grunted.

"He's just a teenager," Julie said reassuring herself as much as Tom. "I'm sure you were a nightmare for your parents when you were in high school."

"If he's getting too much for you to handle, he could come live with Christy and me for a while."

"No," Julie snapped.

"It was just a thought."

"No."

"I could help him with football, maybe increase his chances of getting into a good college program and making the pros."

"Pete lives with me."

Alan McGhee sat on a canvas lawnchair on his front porch reading a novel, his injured leg up on a second, red canvas chair, a blue plastic ice pack wrapped around his knee and held in place with black Velcro straps.

"How long do you have to do that?" Julie asked as she came up the stone steps after a day at work. She had spotted Alan as she turned into her driveway.

"Ten minutes every hour until hell freezes over," he said with a grin.

"Recovery can be slow."

Macduff emerged from a corner of the porch where he had been curled on his tartan cushion. He reached the end of his leash, which was tied around the balustrade and half-growled even as his tail whipped back and forth.

"Hello, Macduff," Julie said.

The terrier growled and let out a powerful bark.

"Oh, Mac, settle down," Alan said. "You know Julie."

With some wariness, Julie held her hand down to the terrier, who sniffed it, then, tail swishing, reared up on his hind legs and shadow boxed with his front paws. Julie scratched him behind the ears.

"Sit down, please."

Julie sat on a cushioned bench that ran along the back of the wide, sheltered porch. She could smell flowers in the air and a hint of the sea.

"I meant to apologize for the other day at the drug store," Julie began, saying something she had been practicing in her mind for days. "I was a little under the weather and didn't feel like talking about it."

"No problem. Everyone has their off days."

Julie nodded, relieved.

They sat in companionable silence as Macduff, the relationship with Julie reestablished, circled several times, scratched at the red tartan of his cushion and settled back down on his snug bed. His black eyes remained open as he surveyed his porch, his yard and his street.

Alan laid his novel, *Crime and Punishment*, on a low metal table beside his chair, shifted in his seat and, glaring at his knee, said, "I think I could build a new knee from spare parts in the time this one's taking to heal."

"Knees are pretty complex," Julie said, happy to move on from the unfortunate incident at the drug store.

"How complex can they be? They support your weight and bend as needed."

"Trust me, they're complex. I hate to boast, but I've seen them from the inside."

"So have I, unfortunately not under as sterile conditions as you probably have."

"Probably not," Julie conceded, blanching at the thought of the scenes Alan must have witnessed in combat.

"I'm sure my United States Military Academy at West Point bachelors of engineering degree prepared me well to build a nice, structurally sound and resilient knee," Alan said, sounding just pompous enough to be funny. "Some nice strong titanium alloy to forge the joint, and..."

"The knee is one of the most complex joints in the body," Julie warned with a smile. "If I remember correctly from medical school; four bones, eight ligaments, and constructed to allow flexion, extension, slight medial and lateral rotation, as well as special locking and unlocking."

"Locking and unlocking? It's a joint, not a doorknob."

Julie laughed.

"Can I get you a drink of something?"

"I think I better get the drinks," she said, eyeing his knee. "But, no thanks, I'm fine."

He looked over at her as she leaned back against the house's ochre adobe wall, stretching her legs out into the sunlight. She felt the rough, cool wall of the house through her blouse as if she lay on a pebbly beach.

Noticing his stare, she asked, "What?"

"Just wondering."

"What?"

"How well I know you."

She smiled and tried to discern where his comment was leading.

"If I don't know you well enough, I won't say anything," he said.

"And if you know me well?" Julie let the corners of her lips turn up and her eyes narrow as she tilted her head toward her right shoulder to look, she hoped, engaging, flirtatious and a touch mysterious.

"If I know you well, I'd ask if you're feeling okay?"

"I just had a bug, that's all," Julie said with as much of a note of finality as she could manage without sounding rude.

He looked far from convinced.

"I'm fine. Really. Why?" she asked, looking away across the yard and up the street toward her house. She wondered what Pete was doing. Was he home yet or still at school? She hoped he had be-haved at football practice today; at least the coach hadn't called her.

"I haven't seen you jogging in weeks," Alan said, his voice even and calm; not the least accusing.

"I've been busy."

He rushed on, "You look pale, you've lost weight, you have enough prescription drugs in your medicine cabinet to stock a pharmacy, and I see your light on in the middle of the night."

"You're an observant neighbor."

"When you command 120 18-year-olds prone to finding what-ever trouble is within 20 clicks of their position and then getting into said trouble, you learn to be observant."

"Does that include patrolling the streets of a residential neigh-borhood in the middle of the night?"

"I have explicit orders from my physio Jihadist to exercise my knee for increasing periods each day, and Macduff needs exercise."

Julie glanced down at the somnolent, diminutive, 20-pound dog. "Don't walk him too far, his legs already look like they've been worn down to the nubs."

"He's a great walker; determined. He just likes walking in the cool of the night." Alan reached down, patted Macduff and turned back to Julie. "Well?"

"Well what?"

"Well, how are you?"

She looked at him, meeting his dark eyes and said, "I'm fine. Just writing a lot. Working on a book."

"That's great. I didn't know you wrote novels. I have an old Academy buddy who writes thrillers. Military adventures with high-tech weaponry, nuclear-armed Islamic terrorists and fearless Amer-ican special ops heroes."

"Published?"

"Five novels. He retired a Major and moved to North Carolina to write; low cost of living and a mild climate."

"Sounds like a wonderful retirement." Julie struggled to keep the jealousy at the thought of publishing five novels out of her voice.

"He likes it." Alan looked over at her, held her eyes with his gaze and said with a disarming grin, "Get some rest. You can't fin-ish writing a book if you're dead."

*The greatest test of courage on earth
is to bear defeat without losing heart.*

—Robert Ingersoll, US statesman,
1833-1899

October

"You missed your God-damn tackle," Joe Cain accused Pete.

"Bullshit," Pete shot back, glaring at the broad-shouldered line-backer after the Spartans' first loss of the season. The locker room was crowded with players changing after their hard-fought defeat. The whip whip of adhesive tape being unwound mixed with the clatter, clicks and thuds of 60 sweating and exhausted boys stripping off grass- and blood-stained pads, cleats and jerseys. Several of the boys stifled tears at the loss while a couple slumped against walls and openly sobbed.

"If coach had me in, they wouldn't have made a yard on that play, let alone fucking 12," Cain said.

"If coach had you in, you wouldn't have known which play we were running. Learn the god-damn playbook before you start boasting how good you think you are."

"I'm a damn sight better than you. There's a reason they don't let girls play football."

"Say that again, you Texas cow-fucker," Pete yelled, his rage-contorted face inches away from Cain's. Pete was tired and weak from fasting for Yom Kippur the day before, but there was no way he was going to take this crap from Cain.

"Your tits are bigger than that fine pair on Jayden's piece of T and A."

Using a short, punishing punch learned long ago during child-hood Taekwondo classes, Pete's right fist connected with Cain's stomach. Cain gasped and doubled over. As he did so, Pete grabbed Cain's left arm and spun him around, yanking the hand up Cain's back to the breaking point.

"Enough!"

Still holding Cain's left hand up to his shoulder, Pete's eyes flicked over to see Coach Paukenan in the doorway.

"Let him go, Tomlinson or you'll be warming the bench with your ass the rest of the season."

It was 3:30 a.m. when Julie's cell sounded. Peering out from under her pillow, which had ended up on top of her head after her attempts to alleviate a throbbing headache, she felt blindly for the cell on her bedside table. Without looking in the dark, she flipped it open.

"MVA; three critical cases," the calm, precise woman at the on-call service reported. "SVU rolled over and all three have trauma to the head, neck and spine."

"I'm on my way."

With regret, Julie rolled out of bed and slipped into her clothes, which she kept on her bedside table for just such calls. She made a quick stop in the bathroom and in less than five minutes was out the door and climbing into her neon yellow VW Bug as she took stock of her aching head, sore throat and a giddy feeling in her chest.

As she pulled out onto the dark, deserted residential street, her stomach grumbled. She should have grabbed a bagel on the way out the door, but it was too late now. Three people needed immedi-ate neurosurgical attention.

She had gone three blocks when her stomach grumbled again. Before she had gone another block it started to roil and boil without pause. After a dozen blocks she realized that she needed to use the bathroom, now. It was only 20 minutes to the hospital, but it seemed a million miles away as her stomach demanded immediate attention.

She had to get to the hospital. Fighting to ignore her stomach and control her bowels, she focused on driving, but hit a red light. Nothing was coming, but she waited, and waited, and waited. She had to use a bathroom, soon, now. She wasn't going to make it to the hospital. She wiggled in the car seat, praying the discomfort and need to go would pass. It did not.

Sweating, she gritted her teeth to control the pain in her stomach. Wincing, she spotted a gas station across the street. Rubbing her stomach to ease the pain, the instant the light changed she roared across the empty intersection and turned into the well-lit station.

She was out of her car and standing before the Hispanic attendant in his bulletproof cubicle before her car had stopped rocking.

"Bathroom, please," she asked, inhaling to suppress the pain and the urge to go.

The bespectacled and pony-tailed attendant reached back and grabbed a key attached to a piece of inch-thick, white plastic pipe the length of a ruler.

"You have to be a customer," he said, holding the key tantalizingly close, but on his side of the thick, scarred and scuffed security glass.

"I'll buy a candy bar as soon as I come out," Julie promised, wishing he would just hand it over as she shifted from foot to foot.

With a put-upon sigh the attendant pushed the key through the slot to Julie, who grabbed it and sprinted for the restroom.

The diarrhea had been intensifying. She was taking more anti-diarrheals, which dehydrated her, causing headaches no matter how much she drank. The diuretics for her hypertension only increased her dehydration. Worse, the anti-diarrheals were losing their effectiveness. Given the painful side effects on her stomach and head, the recurring olfactory hallucinations and hypertension, not to mention the constant metallic taste in her mouth, she would have quit taking the trial drugs if not for the fact that her writing was rolling along as if her hand was being guided by the Bard himself. She had to keep taking the drugs until she finished her novel, which, if things continued going as well as they had been, would be within a month. The stomach trouble, headaches and occasional dizziness slowed her writing since they made it difficult to concentrate, let alone sit and write, but come what may, she would get her novel done—soon. She had to.

She emerged from the restroom 10 minutes later, drained and weak. Looking down at her hands, she realized that they were shaking. Returning the key to the attendant, who shot her an expectant look, she bought an Oh Henry! and was about to hurry on to the hospital when she realized she needed to go again right away. This time there would be no possibility of waiting even a moment.

"I need the key again, please," Julie told the attendant, wishing she had never left the bathroom.

The attendant lowered his pony-tailed head and looked up at her over his black-framed glasses. He looked as if he was appraising a potential thief.

"I had some bad seafood," Julie lied. She wondered how he could suspect that a single white woman driving a neon yellow VW Beetle would stop by to scribble graffiti in a gas station toilet at 3 am on a Tuesday night.

The attendant considered and then with a sour look pushed the key back through the slot.

When Julie left the bathroom the second time, she felt even weaker, more nauseous, and had to concentrate on walking to avoid stumbling. Her head was pounding with an intense headache that bordered on what was called a thunderclap headache; a symptom of a brain tumor. She knew she didn't have a brain tumor, but it sure felt like the headaches some of her patients described when they had a tumor.

Concentrating to control the pain, she resolved to get to the hospital and evaluate the three MVA patients. They needed her. She was on call. It was her responsibility. She had to do it. She had to get there. But as she sat in her VW, willing her body to cooperate, she realized she could not do it. The sweat that had bathed her body had turned into a clammy glaze of moisture covering her skin. Her hands tingled and when she held them out before her eyes, they shook worse than before. She was far from being in condition to give someone a shot, let alone perform a craniotomy or spinal tap, if any such procedure was needed. It would be irresponsible for her to operate in such a condition.

Giving in, she reached for her purse and, checking its contents, swore. She had left her cell on the bedside table. Her persistent headaches were affecting her ability to perform the most simple tasks.

She spotted a phone booth on the corner, but even from where she sat she could see that the phone had been removed, a victim of the increasing diffusion of cell phones. She was closer to home than to the hospital, so she started her car and raced home. She just made it. Rushing inside to the bathroom, she finished her urgent business there and then called one of the other neurosurgeons.

"You're sick?" Ken Yu asked, far from happy at being awoken during one of his off nights. "Why didn't you tell the service when they paged you?"

"I thought I'd be able to make it."

"The service just called me, looking for you."

"I left my cell at home by accident."

"I thought you were at home."

"I am, I was, I started to go to the hospital and couldn't make it."

"Why didn't you tell the service you were sick? Since they called you one of the patients slid into a coma."

"I Still Haven't Found What I'm Looking For"

—U2, *The Joshua Tree*, 1987

After school Pete was usually at football practice or home alone until his mom finished work, but not today. Today was a rare day when there was no football practice, so today Amanda lay against him, naked under the sheets of his double bed.

"Maybe we can try again in a little while," she said, rubbing him along his muscular thighs.

"My mom will be home soon," Pete said, furious with himself. Rolling onto his side, he looked down at his girlfriend, her blonde hair splayed out around her head, her eyes wide and seductive as she looked up at him. He pulled the sheet down to admire her pert, round breasts, which without fail fired his passion. Blood had reddened her chest. Her nipples were erect and hard. She was ready, but he was not. He ran his hand under and around the nearer breast, leaning down to kiss it: nothing. Anger boiled within him.

"I'm sure you're just tired," she said, kissing him. "It happens."

"How would you know?" he snapped, regretting the words as soon as he said them.

She sat up and pulled the sheet up to her neck. Her glare was more forceful than any words. She had gone from passion of one kind to passion of another in the time it took him to say those four spiteful words.

"I'm sorry," he said, his voice low. He was sorry, but also furious that he had lost his temper.

"That was not very nice." She slid out of bed, giving Pete a moment to admire her long, tanned legs, and started dressing, her back to him.

"Amanda, don't go." He reached for her, but she slipped away as she pulled on her tight jeans with some wiggling, which jiggled her breasts provocatively. Pete noticed, but it did nothing for him.

"You're mom will be home soon, remember?" The frozen edge in her voice matched her rigid body language.

"Don't be like that. I said I was sorry. I was…I was just mad we couldn't do it." The rage subsided as suddenly as it had arisen.

She snapped on her black bra and adjusted it, emphasizing for Pete what he was missing.

"Having sex with you is so great, I hate missing a chance," he said.

"You don't mean that."

"I do," but even as he said the words, he realized he really didn't care that much. Football, working out and keeping his grades at a Mom-acceptable B level filled his life right now. Amanda was hot, but his interest in her had been declining. He was just too busy and too tired most of the time to care about sex, or maybe he was just tired of her. When they had started dating the year before, they had done it several times a week. Now they rarely made the time to arrange to be alone once a month. And when they did, he found it routine, even boring.

"If you like sex with me so much, then you should be nicer to me," Amanda said, her voice no warmer than before.

"I am." The rage was building again.

Pulling on her maroon blouse, she spun around, her long, straight hair flying around her. "You snap at me, you spend all your time working out, and you spend two hours out on the porch at Bruce's party with that butch, Adina."

"She's not a butch."

"She is."

"She's…" Pete saw the trap he had constructed for himself too late.

"She's what? Pretty? Sexy?"

"We were just talking," he said, tired of the verbal combat.

"I wish you talked to me that much or am I only good for sex?"

Pete sighed, hanging his head as he sat on the bed, the sheet bunched up around his waist. "I have to train or I'll never make it to college, let alone the pros. If we want to have the life we've talked about, I have to."

"You could spare some time for me. What with football, basketball and baseball, I never see you."

"That's it, isn't it?" he said, raising his head to glare at her.

"What?"

"You want me to fail so I'll have more time for you. You don't want me to ever make it to the pros."

"Why on Earth wouldn't I?" she asked, her eyebrows arched in amazement.

"You're afraid I'll have a babe in every town and I'll dump you."

"Maybe you should. I obviously don't interest you much any-more—to go out with, talk to or in bed."

Pete's rage surged again at her verbal attack and he spat back, "Maybe you're right. I hold a girl's hand, I get a hard-on, but with you naked, nothing. Maybe I just need a better-looking girlfriend."

"Good luck finding anyone who'll take you, you bastard," she screamed and stormed out, crying.

He leaned back, bouncing his head off the wood headboard and with each thunk he yelled, "Damn it! Damn it! Damn it!"

An hour later, he wondered what had ever come over him.

"What's wrong?" Pete asked his mom as she came in that evening from work.

"I'm fine," she said. "Just a little tired."

Pete looked at her. Her eyes had coal-dark pouches beneath them. The lustrous hair that usually framed her face was dull, life-less and dry. Her erect posture had become a stoop. "You need to take better care of yourself, Mom."

"I'll be fine," she said as she slouched down onto the sofa. "I just need a little rest."

"I'll get dinner," Pete offered. He felt like being nice to someone after the way he had treated Amanda. He thought about calling

Amanda, but didn't know what to say, assuming she'd even take his call.

"Thanks, Pete, but my stomach's been a little upset. I think I'll pass."

Pete looked down at her on the sofa. Was she going to be okay? She pushed herself so hard that although she rarely got sick, when she did, it was bad and prolonged. "Can I get you anything?"

"A new body?" his mom asked with a grin.

"You only get one, so take care of it," Pete said, no hint of levity in his voice.

"Yes, doctor."

"Starters for tomorrow night are Joe Cain and Pete Tomlinson," Coach told the three linebackers after practice Thursday afternoon.

"Tough break, Jayden," Pete told his teammate as they sauntered back across the playing fields toward the locker room, sweat-soaked, exhausted and aching from a grueling practice. Barrels of ice awaited them to assuage the aches and pains in as much of their bodies as would fit in the 50-gallon plastic barrels.

"I missed two tackles last week and I've been fighting a cold," Jayden explained without even a hint that either was an excuse for not starting for the first time this season. "I'll start next week, and I'll put on a highlights show if coach puts me in as tight end tomorrow night."

Pete nodded. Jayden was always optimistic, especially about himself.

The sophomore safety Manny Ortiz called to Pete as he rushed past, "Coach promised he'd get me in for a couple of plays."

"That's great, Manny," Pete said, grinning at the excited safety.

"I got another letter," Jayden said, swinging his helmet at his side as he walked, "Wisconsin. Full scholarship if I keep my stats up."

"Sweet."

"You?"

"USC, Michigan, Illinois, Minnesota, Arkansas, Oregon, and Miami are all interested."

"Full scholarships?"

"They can't promise, but like you, if I keep my numbers up, I've got a free ride."

"Keep beating Cain and you're set."

"Not a problem," Pete said, full of confidence.

"And," Jayden said, "Next week I'll beat his black ass too."

The members of the Medical Case Review Board were some of the most senior physicians on Mount Hermon's medical staff. Their CVs ran to more than 100 pages each, with hundreds of published articles, and three dozen lucrative patents between them. They had logged thousands of hours in the OR. They had been to the best medical schools, interned and completed residencies at Mayo, Cleveland Clinic, the University of Chicago, Oxford, Cambridge, and Johns Hopkins. They earned in the top one percent of the American population. They were smart, driven and competitive, with no patience for mistakes. When lives were at stake, mistakes meant people died.

Julie glanced at Andrew Baxter, who served on the board, and hoped his subtle nod was a sign of hope, unlike his performance during the SAE Committee review of her study. Even so, she felt far from optimistic.

"Why didn't you appear for the call?" Dr. Peter Weinstein, Chair of Imaging asked. With pale blue eyes, a shock of white hair and wire-rimmed spectacles, he looked like a kindly grandfather, but Julie had seen him lose his temper once—luckily not at her—and it was not something she ever wished to see again.

"I was ill," Julie said. Sitting at the long conference table with all eyes on her, she felt like a prisoner in the dock for a capital crime.

"Why didn't you call another neurosurgeon?" Dr. Randy Johnson asked. Chair of Orthopaedics, he was tall and thin with a predatory hawk-like face that had terrified more than one resident.

"I thought I could make it to the hospital, but when I tried I couldn't. When I realized I couldn't make it, I was going to call Ken Yu to cover for me but I had forgotten my cell on my bedside table. I had a severe headache."

"A headache?" Johnson asked, the Texas twang in his voice becoming more pronounced.

"Yes. I wasn't thinking clearly."

"Not a quality we look for in our neurosurgeons," Baxter commented looking straight at Julie.

Julie fell silent. So much for his support.

"So your explanation is that you had a headache, tried to come in, could not, and forgot your cell to call someone to cover for you?" Johnson asked.

"Yes." Julie could see little reason to mention the stomach ache given the cold reception the headache had received. "Once I reached home, I called Ken at once."

"By which time one of the patients had slipped into a coma," Weinstein observed, peering at her over his spectacles, as if inspecting an especially odious specimen of cancer he'd discovered on an MRI.

Julie remained silent. What could she say?

The six physicians on the board glanced at each other. Gentlemanly, white-haired Dr. Kanavou, Chief of Staff, asked her to step outside while they discussed the case.

Three minutes later she was back before them.

"It is the decision of this board," Kanavou intoned in his baritone, "that your privileges at Mount Hermon Medical Center be revoked for one week. You made a serious error in judgment and put a patient at risk of a significant adverse event, not to mention exposing yourself and the Medical Center to a potential lawsuit. Any repetition of an incident like this and you will lose your privileges permanently. Understood?"

Julie walked to the car, drained and dejected, but relieved that she had not been terminated. From habit, she checked her voicemail on her cell. Hsu, her research assistant, had left a message at 2 am the night before. Like many researchers, he worked late hours, offset by coming into the lab late each morning. She should have checked her messages that morning, but her mind had been engulfed by worries about what would happen at the Case Review meeting.

"Julie, Hsu," she heard as the message played. "A pharmacist came to pick up the clinical trial drugs. Kanavou authorized their transfer to inpatient use, but the pharmacist said some of the drugs are missing."

The distance between insanity and genius
is measured only by success.

—Bruce Feirstein, US screenwriter, b. 1956

Three days after the board meeting revoked Julie's privileges for a week, she sat in a plush, leather chair in Andrew Baxter's corner office. A legend in neurosurgery, Baxter had invented a dozen different types of improved shunts, cauterizing tools, surgical procedures and treatments for brain tumors. He was the leader in one of the most hyper-competitive fields in the world. The United States has as many neurosurgeons as fighter pilots, but for all the flash and style of fighter pilots, neurosurgeons are much better paid and have far more lives in their hands than fighter pilots—at least during peacetime.

"This is the worst part of my job," Baxter began.

Terror coursed through Julie as she stared vacantly at a sextant that sat in a weathered wood box on the corner of Baxter's expansive desk. As a neurosurgeon, every day Baxter told families that their loved one was dead or never going to be the same person they had been before some trauma or tragedy struck. If this was the worst part of his job, what was he about to tell her?

"I understand you've admitted taking the pharmaceuticals for your trial from my lab?" he asked as if commenting on the surgery schedule.

"Yes," she said, resisting the urge to correct him and say, 'My lab.'

"Why?" Baxter asked.

Julie met his gaze. There was nothing to lose in telling the truth, since the alternative was to be labeled a thief. "My clinical trial showed that the drug combination led to increased creativity."

"As I understand it, the findings merely suggested that correlation." He did not have to say that a suggestion of a correlation was years of research away from showing whether the drug combination caused an increase in creativity.

She cut to the heart of the matter. "I wanted to determine if my creativity would increase under the drug regimen."

"And whether it increased the risk of TIA and stroke, as well as," he said, flipping open a dark blue manila folder on his desk before reading, "liver problems, osteoporosis, GI irritation, dry mouth, headache, hypertension, hallucinations, and who knows what else?"

"I don't believe the risks are significant for someone my age."

"Have the drugs been tested on non-geriatric subjects?"

"No."

"Therefore you have no way of knowing the risks for someone your age. Given such unknown risks, why in God's name did you take them?"

"I want to be a novelist."

His look of surprise could not have been greater if she had admitted to a secret desire to be a moose.

"Then write a bloody novel," he said, his eyes narrow, his mouth an uncomprehending scowl of derision.

"I've tried. Not much luck publishing."

"Try again."

"I have."

"Then maybe you should stick to being a God-damn neurosurgeon."

Baxter's well-scrubbed index finger fidgeted with a loose piece of paper in the file on his desk. He let out a short breath as if to cleanse himself of the mention of becoming a novelist and asked, "Did the drugs make you miss the emergent call in which a patient

slid into a coma and almost died, a result only averted by Boardman, who happened to be at the hospital?"

"Yes. I was rather ill."

"From the drugs you were taking?"

"Yes."

"That was extremely irresponsible."

"I thought I could make it in."

"Apparently you thought wrong." He shut the file and looked
across at her again. Running his hand through his short gray hair,
he sighed. "I don't have any choice, Julie. The hospital can't allow
physicians, no matter how gifted, to steal, let alone miss a critical
case when they're on call."

"The board already suspended me and I will pay for the drugs."

"That's beside the point," Baxter said, his voice, for the first
time rising to fill the spacious office. "Do you realize how damag-
ing it would be to the hospital if it became known that one of our
doctors, let alone a neurosurgeon, was taking drugs that had been
part of a discontinued clinical trial in which a patient died, and
because she was taking those drugs, she missed a critical trauma
emergency call? Not only your judgment would be called into serious question, but so would mine and the entire hospital administration's for hiring you, let alone for keeping you on staff."

Julie managed to nod. The ache behind her eyes, which seemed
constant in recent weeks, spiked with a sudden intensity that made
her narrow her eyes in a wince.

"Why on earth did you do this?" Baxter asked, bewildered.

"I want to be a novelist."

"I would think saving someone's life is a little more important
than writing a God-damn novel."

"I didn't think the two were mutually exclusive."

"Apparently the way you do them, they are."

Julie looked over at Baxter's vanity wall of degrees, awards and
publications. She looked back at him and said, "If you could take
a drug that would help you discover a cure for malignant brain tumors, help millions of people and win a Nobel Prize, wouldn't you
take the drug even if it meant risking your own health?"

Baxter exhaled through his nose in a snort, but when Julie continued to wait for an answer, he sighed and admitted, "Not that it

relates at all to your case, since there's little evidence your drugs increase creativity, but if it was going to work—maybe."

With just the hint of a smile, Julie looked at him, having, she thought, won a point.

"If you were so damn sure of it, you could have run a clinical trial to test your hypothesis about the drugs and creativity."

"How could I, with one trial already stopped?"

"Then the drugs are too risky."

"Some things are worth the risk."

"Nothing's worth the risk if it means someone dies when they weren't facing imminent death."

"The patients in my study had Alzheimer's and were geriatric," Julie said, realizing even as she said it how weak an argument it was.

"Geriatric, yes; on death's door, no."

"The drugs were effective."

Baxter stared at her, far from understanding.

"My writing greatly improved."

"Says you."

"Says a literary agent and a publisher. They want to publish my novel."

"Congratulations," Baxter said, the word dripping with sarcasm. "Whatever is happening with your literary endeavors, I am responsible for overseeing your surgical endeavors." He paused, leaned back and then set his elbows on his desk to face her full on. "I am sorry, especially since I'm the one who brought you aboard, but I am forced by your recent behavior to suspend you." He paused and continued in a business-like tone, "You will no longer have OR privileges. You will no longer see patients in clinic at this hospital and you will no longer have access to the labs."

"For how long?" Julie asked, knowing this suspension would be longer than a week.

Baxter drummed his short, stubby fingers, daily scrubbed in the OR to a pale white, on the edge of his desk. "The Committee on Medical Ethics will meet at the end of the month and then the Medical Supervisory and Administrative Committee will convene to decide based on their recommendations how to proceed. I'm sure the Medical Case Review Board will also have input into the decision about how long to suspend you—or whether to pursue another course."

Julie didn't need to ask what the other courses might be: dismissal.

When Julie arrived home there was a phone message from Sylvia, Baxter's management assistant asking Julie to please return all the drugs from her clinical trial immediately. Julie swore and dropped her bag on the kitchen table. It was just like Baxter to have his assistant do his dirty work. For those below him, Baxter had the social skills of a feudal despot. A few years before a researcher and the Neurosurgical Institute's grant writer had written a grant proposal that was awarded $2.5 million from the National Institutes of Health. The CEO of Mount Hermon sent an enormous flower bouquet to Baxter, since he was head of the lab that had been awarded the grant, even though he had been only tangentially involved in developing the grant proposal. Baxter sent the flowers to the researcher, with a brief note of thanks. The researcher planned to take the flowers home to his wife but that afternoon, just as he was about to leave, Baxter sent his assistant Sylvia over to pick up the flowers. They had just been on loan for the day. Apoplectic, the researcher was now a principle investigator at Vanderbilt University, producing dozens of research papers a year supported by not one, but two NIH grants.

Julie stalked off to her bathroom and, yanking open the medicine cabinet, glared at the row of plastic bottles containing the drugs from her trial. She considered keeping some so she could keep taking the drugs a few more days. She could get further along on her novel, but if Baxter found out that she hadn't returned all of the drugs, he would terminate her for certain.

As she stormed out of her house, a plastic bag full of drugs jangling in her hand, she almost ran into Alan McGhee on the front steps.

"What's wrong?" he asked.

"I was sick, missed a call at work, got suspended, and my head and stomach feel like they'll never be well again," Julie roared, losing her temper.

"They suspend you if you're sick?" Alan asked in disbelief.

"They do if you're taking drugs from your discontinued clinical trial, which made you sick, which then made you miss the call."

Alan stared at her. "Why, I don't understand…"

"There's not much to understand," she snapped.

"Why were you taking the drugs?"

Turning on her heel, she sped back inside and returned a moment later clutching a sheaf of paper. "So I could write this," she said, thrusting it at him.

"I still don't understand."

"The drugs increase creativity, so I can write better."

"But they make you sick?"

"Yes."

"Seriously sick?"

"Not yet."

"Not yet?" he asked, bewildered. "How sick?"

"One patient had a TIA, and another had a stroke and died."

"You were taking drugs that might kill you?" Alan asked, shocked.

"Yes."

"Why?"

"Read that," Julie said, jabbing a finger at the papers she had given him. "I have to go." She strode around him, scrambled into her car, slammed the door, and sped off, leaving a shocked and confused Alan on her doorstep clutching the first three chapters of her novel manuscript.

Don't be afraid to give up the good
to go for the great.

—John D. Rockefeller

It was a warm October night and the sell-out crowd was on its feet. With only 18 seconds left in the first half, the Carson Graham Highlanders were pressing to score against the Santa Maria Spartans. With the game tied, Pete and his teammates were desperate to keep the Highlanders out of the end zone and allow them only a field goal, if that.

On the Spartans' 8-yard line, the Highlanders could in all likelihood run two pass plays in 18 seconds. One run would eat up the clock. Expecting a pass, the Spartans coach sent in a blitz. Pete shifted over to the strong side, glancing over to see Cain move closer to the line to blitz. Manny Ortiz was in at safety. He wouldn't have been if one of the Spartans' starting safeties hadn't torn an ACL on the previous play. Pete checked Manny's positioning; perfect.

The Highlander quarterback came up to center and scanned the field.

"Down!"

Pete moved up to the line. His eyes flitted back and forth between the Highlander backfield—a one running back set—and the two wide receivers on his side of the field covered by Manny and

Sanchez, the other Spartans safety. Manny better do his job. He was good enough to cover his receiver, but he would be excited, nervous and anxious, any of which could lead to a game-losing mistake.

"Set!"

Pete saw the Highlander running back wipe his hands on his thighs.

"Hike!"

Nothing.

"Hike!" The center snapped the ball hard into the quarterback's waiting hands.

The lines crashed into each other. Cain sliced through a gap, rushing for the quarterback as the Highlander line began to disintegrate. Rushing around the end of the line, Pete was about to race into the pocket to beat Cain to the quarterback when he sensed something wrong. The Highlander line had held all night and now they collapsed?

Glancing left he spotted the lone running back fading back and out, away from the center of the play; a screen pass.

Pete wheeled left even as the quarterback turned and lofted the ball out to the running back, over the onrushing Spartans tackle and end. The two receivers had shifted in to block for the back as he caught the ball. The back streaked up field; eight yards from six points and the lead.

As Adina had taught him, Pete kept his legs square and vertical as he raced after the running back. As he crossed the five, Pete stretched out and grabbed the back around the waist just as one of the back's blockers drove Manny Ortiz onto his back on the turf.

Pete hung on as the back twisted and turned to break free. Pete's left hand slid up and under the back's collar. Pete grabbed the back's shoulder pads from the inside. Before he could be called for a necktie penalty, Pete brought the back down over backwards on the two-yard line.

"God damn you," the back roared at Pete as they tumbled into a heap.

"Just doing my job, asshole," Pete said. "Same as I'll do every time you touch the fucking ball."

Bouncing back to his feet, Pete started to jog back to the huddle before he realized the half was over. The slow-developing Highlander screen had eaten up the remaining 18 seconds. As Pete turned to trot to the dressing room, he felt an odd sensation in his throat. He took another step. His heart sputtered and bounced all around in his chest. It felt as if there was an alien inside him, fighting to escape. A crushing pain struck deep in his chest.

Pete put his hands on the grass-stained knees of his football pants and focused on breathing, trying to calm his heart as he winced at the pain. Even as he did, his body shook all over. It was a warm night, with the Santa Ana's blowing hot, dry air from the desert inland, which, he thought, must be why he felt so awful. He should have drunk more water—but, he had been.

The pain passed as suddenly as it had struck, but the bizarre feeling continued.

"You okay?"

Pete looked up. Manny Ortiz, the sophomore safety, stood before him.

"Fine," Pete grunted.

"Thanks for saving that play."

"No problem."

Pete steeled his nerves and forced himself to walk off the field with Manny, across the cinder track and down the cool, dark tunnel into the dressing room. Once inside, he barely noticed the horde of other players, drinking water or being administered IV fluid as they slumped on the floor, on benches and against lockers or the concrete walls. Pete collapsed onto a bench.

Pete's heart bounced around. He felt as if he had lost control of his body. He grabbed a water from a passing freshman waterboy and chugged it down, dropping the empty bottle on the floor. He was in a panic. It took all his resolve not to scream for help. What was happening? Was he going to die?

"You alright?" Jayden asked, eyeing Pete with a worried expression. Benched, Jayden's uniform was a pristine white and green.

"Just hot," Pete said, trying to sound normal, but gasping as he spoke. He realized he was panting.

Jayden stared at Pete and yelled, "Rox, Tomlinson needs you."

"You okay, Pete?" the trainer asked as she crouched before him, her eyes skimming over him from head to cleats. In her twenties, Rox was a physiotherapist with first-aid training who worked for the team part-time and dreamed of one day working for the Philadelphia Eagles, her home-town team.

"I'm alright," Pete said, casting a glare at Jayden. "Just hot. Be fine as soon as I get my breath back."

Rox stuck a thermometer in his mouth without preamble and checked his pulse, taking it in his neck, since his wrists were wrapped with layers of grass- and blood-stained tape.

"Your temperature is a little high," she said a minute later. "Your heart beat's irregular. You ever had heart trouble?"

As the rest of the team guzzled sports drinks, stretched or were praised, berated or lectured by various coaches, Pete said, "No, never."

With the greatest relief, he felt his heart beat normally again.

"We could try some IV fluids, but I think I should call an ambulance," Rox said, starting to rise.

Pete caught her tanned arm. "Check my pulse again. It's back to normal."

Rox hesitated. When Pete kept clutching her forearm, she said, "Alright. We'll get some fluid into you. I'm going to recommend you sit out the rest of the game."

"No, don't. I'm fine. I'm playing great."

Looking far from convinced, Rox listened to his heart again and reported a minute later, "You're heart seems back to normal, but I'm still going to talk to Coach."

"I can play."

"I'll give you an IV, but you aren't going to play."

"I can play."

"It's just half a game, Pete," she said, sitting down on her haunches before him to look him in the eyes. "I want to make sure you're completely well before you get out there again." She smiled to lessen Pete's disappointment. It didn't work.

Money is coined liberty.

—Fyodor Dostoevsky

Julie arose the next morning after a restless night, hoping Pete felt better. She had suffered through vivid dreams of Pete growing into a giant before her eyes, bursting through the ceiling of his room and destroying first their house, then the neighborhood and finally the world. She had awoken at 2:25 a.m. disoriented, shaking and filmed with sweat. By morning the vivid dreams had receded and she had at least managed to get a couple of hours of sleep.

She opened Pete's bedroom door and found him snoring amid a tangle of sheets. She frowned at what looked like a new pair of sneakers on the floor, resting in a pristine box. With an indulgent shake of her head, she thought that Pete would buy anything that caught his eye.

Slipping over to look down at him, she still found it amazing that such a huge boy—a man—had been her little baby. She had once been able to hold him in the crook of her arm, swing him around at arm's length to his delight, and had been responsible for everything he did. Not anymore.

Staring down at him, she noted that his color was better. She had forced him to drink a hydration solution the night before when they arrived home, which had helped. She pulled a blanket up over him to ward off the morning chill, such as there was in West Los Angeles in October, and slipped back out of his room to the kitchen.

It was Saturday and unbidden she thought that she wasn't on call this weekend. Then it struck her that she had been suspended. She hadn't told Tom. She wanted to tell him so he would hear it from her, not from someone else. She should have told him last night, but Christy had been there and the last person she wanted to tell was Christy. Julie despised Christy; all body and no brains, except for business. Christy bought and sold things on E-bay and made more money than Tom, and Tom made a good living. For all her belief in empiricism, such things made Julie believe in luck; how else do you explain the success of people you despise?

Thinking of money, Julie went over her finances. With the suspension, her paychecks had stopped. She had some money saved besides her retirement accounts, which carried substantial penalties for early withdrawal. If she watched every dime, she should have enough for a few months, six at the most, which should see them through the suspension. She avoided thinking about what would happen if she was terminated. She had read that you should have six months of income saved for an emergency, but even if you did, six months was an awfully short period in which to find another job. Finding another job would be difficult, if not impossible without recommendations from Mount Hermon, and how could she explain her sudden departure from one of the finest medical centers in the country?

Chasing such thoughts from her mind, she considered going jogging, but her head ached and her stomach was still sore. Now that she was off the drugs, the side effects should soon subside.

With her mind turning to writing, she thought about the creativity the trial drugs had ignited in her. She was desperate to keep that feeling. She considered writing herself prescriptions for the drugs. The drugs were common. It was the combination that was new. Self-prescribing was frowned upon, even though every physician did it. But if Mount Hermon found out, she would be terminated. She could not risk it. She would write without the drugs every moment she could while the effect of the drugs lasted.

Early the following Sunday morning she walked into her home office and sat down at her laptop on her maple desk. As she had been doing for days, she prayed the effect of the drugs on her creativity would last another day.

She read the prose she had completed the night before and tried to write the next sentence. Nothing came. She reread the previous few paragraphs, thought about the story arc and wrote five sentences. Rereading them, she grimaced; wooden and clunky. She deleted them and tried again. She read the new paragraph. Still far from good, but it would have to do for now. She forged on, struggling with every paragraph, sentence and word.

An hour later, she heard Pete's bathroom door close. She reread what she had written. It was bad. Her head lolled to her chest. She groaned and gathered her courage. British journalist and novelist, Arthur Quiller-Couch called it "murdering your darlings," but if it was no good, it had to go. There was no point trying to publish drivel. She highlighted the page and a half she had just struggled for an hour to write and not giving herself time to change her mind, hit delete.

Her hour's work gone, sitting with her head down, she heard the shower start. What was she going to do? The effect of the drugs had worn off. She was doomed. Wood-Byrd and the publisher had loved the first sample chapters of her novel. They would hate what she was writing now. Even she hated it. Her writing now seemed worse than what she had written before she started taking the drugs. She realized that it was just because what she had written under the influence of the drugs had been so good, but even knowing that she couldn't convince herself that her current writing didn't stink.

With a sigh, she checked her email for lack of anything better to do. She answered a few messages and was about to delete yet another spam email when she stopped. "Cheap Drugs from Canada" read the subject line. Her hand froze with the cursor above the delete button. After considering, she moved the cursor and opened the e-mail.

The ad said they accepted prescriptions from all 50 US states. She could write her own. Would anyone find out? If Mount Hermon requested a list of the prescriptions written under her California license, would it show up if the drugs had been ordered from Canada? Unlikely, given how rarely governments cooperate. Even so, if Mount Hermon discovered that she was still taking the trial drugs, she would lose her job and probably never find another.

She leaned back in her office chair. If she published her novel and it sold well, she would never need to practice medicine again. She had no doubt that Michael Crichton never saw another patient after *The Andromeda Strain* hit the bestseller lists and she doubted Sir Arthur Conan Doyle worried about his practice in Southsea after Sherlock Holmes became the most famous consulting detective in the world.

She could have the drugs shipped to Pete. He used his father's surname, Tomlinson. She had reverted to her maiden name of Stein years ago. That would decrease the chance that anyone would find out. It seemed a tiny risk and the benefits immeasurable. But there was still a risk.

...after puberty the personality develops impetuously and all extraneous intervention becomes odious, tyrannical, insufferable.

—Antonio Gramsci, Italian philosopher, writer and politician, 1891-1937

November

"Pete, dinner!" Julie called from the kitchen. As she turned to pick up a potholder, the floor undulated beneath her feet as if she was surfing on a rolling sea. Grabbing the granite counter edge for support, she almost fell as nausea washed over her. Panic clawed at her, engulfing her mind and body. Then, as quickly as the hallucination struck, it passed. Swallowing bile and breathing hard, Julie regained her composure.

The drugs from Canada had arrived two days before. With the new drug supply, she was writing fabulously again. The side effects from the drugs had already returned, but she was taking various over-the-counter drugs to counteract them. Since she was suspended, she had more time to write and would be able to finish the novel and quit taking the drugs that much sooner.

Minutes later the nausea and hallucination passed. She called, "Pete, dinner!"

She had not heard from the hospital yet. When she called Sylvia to inquire, the management assistant said the decision about Julie's future at Mount Hermon would not be made for another week or so. Worse, Julie hadn't seen Alan since she had thrust her novel chapters at him. She had been on the verge several times of going over to his house to apologize. Each time she concluded that she couldn't defend her actions unless he understood how she felt about writing and, if he didn't like what she had written, there was no chance of him ever understanding. He would think she was a fool; throwing away her medical career for a miniscule chance to become a novelist.

Even so, Julie felt optimistic. Alan would come around. At least he would if he was the man she hoped he was. Her savings should last until even the labyrinthine Mount Hermon decided to reinstate her. And she would publish a novel; that single success would produce a blaze of glory that would cast all her other worries into shadow.

As Julie was about to call again, Pete emerged from his room, spotted the deep fryer and cut-up chicken, carrots, peppers, parsley and zucchini for tempura on the kitchen counter and announced, "I can't eat that stuff."

"Why not?" Julie asked, exasperated and still weak and unsettled from the hallucination. Taking a deep breath to calm herself, she said, "You love tempura."

"I can't eat all that grease."

"We rarely have it."

"I can't."

"Just once won't hurt," Julie said, seeing all her work cutting up the vegetables and chicken into bite-size pieces wasted.

"You just don't understand, Mom," Pete yelled, his face reddening as he gestured at her with his big, tanned hands. "You just don't realize what I have to go through to make it to the pros!"

"I…" Julie began, shocked at her son's sudden anger.

"You're just like Amanda," he screamed. "You don't want me to make it to college, let alone the pros! You want me fat and out of shape!" He spun on his heal and stalked back to his room.

"Pete," Julie called, stunned and reeling.

Pete slammed his bedroom door; the sound reverberating through Julie's aching head.

There are three rules for writing the novel.
Unfortunately, no one knows what they are.

—W. Somerset Maugham, English dramatist
and novelist, 1874-1965

"The two new chapters are fantastic, sublime," Charles Wood-Byrd rhapsodized over the phone one bright, clear morning. "Jonathan Sharpe positively gushed over them like a school girl."

Julie rose from the sofa from where she had been sitting when her agent called and floated over to the back window.

"Jonathan asked me for the tenth time if I was showing the chapters to anyone else," Charles said with a chuckle. "He wants to make certain we don't involve him in a messy and costly bidding war. I had a rather fine opportunity to be involved in one a few weeks ago between two of the big houses. Between you, me, the author and the rather generous publisher, I will say that the final offer topped six figures for a first novel."

"That's wonderful."

"I don't know what he'll offer, but he assured me he'll pay top dollar for the novel as soon as it's finished, as well as a nice marketing campaign to launch it—and you. I could negotiate a contract now, but I think he'll pay even more once he reads the completed novel. He loves each new chapter more than the previous chapter."

Looking out across the backyard at the roses along the back fence of her yard, Julie beamed. "That's fantastic news," she said.

A giant, red dragon rose out of the roses and launched itself, its jaws gaping open revealing scalpel-sharp teeth, straight at Julie. She gasped and staggered back as an inferno of red, yellow and orange flames belched from the dragon's mouth. She fell to the floor, dropping the phone as she scrambled to avoid the fiery blast.

Shaking and with a glaze of cold sweat gilding her skin, she lay on the carpet. Steeling herself, she reached for the phone.

Charles asked, "Julie? Julie, are you alright?"

"Yes, yes," she said, her heart pounding in her ears. "I just stumbled and dropped the phone." She peeked out at the garden: no dragon.

The Friday night crowd wore puffy jackets, scarves and sweatshirts. The Santa Ana's weren't blowing this November night. Instead an ocean breeze from the west brought a pleasant, fall atmosphere to the Spartans' game at East Los Angeles High School.

Pete lined up defensively on third and three. Coach had called a blitz, but the East LA Toros were showing a two-running-back set. Because coach valued Pete's ability to make snap decisions, it was his job to change the defensive scheme if, after lining up, the offense appeared to be running a different play.

Pete yelled the team's code for a run defense, "Tango!" Turning his head to the right and left, he repeated his warning twice to Jayden and all his teammates at the top of his voice. Cain, who coach hadn't selected to play, sulked and seethed on the sidelines.

Just as the quarterback stepped up behind center, Pete's heart missed a beat. From one second to the next, he went from feeling 100 percent to feeling horrible. Faint, nauseous and with an all-encompassing sense of unease bordering on terror, he felt as if every cell in his body was shaking.

"Down!"

Pete struggled to calm his body. His heart raced and skipped beats. He had to get it together. This was a crucial game.

"Set!"

He had to move up to the line. His taped hands fell to his padded thighs. He struggled to get his heart to stop racing, his body to stop shaking. He gasped for air. Nausea washed over him in sickening waves.

"Hike!"

The center hiked the ball. Pete's eyesight blurred. His vision faded to black and white. His world shrank to just his own body. As the play swirled and rushed around him, he fell to his knees. Lightheaded and weak, his body filled with a terror: the terror that his heart was failing him.

No one keeps a secret so well as a child.

—Victor Hugo

"What's your diagnosis?" Julie asked in her most authoritative medical voice at East Los Angeles Memorial Hospital at 2:15 am.

Tom and Christy stood beside her in the hall outside the ER exam room where Pete lay hooked up to an EKG monitor.

"Heart palpitations," the sedate ER doctor, who smelled of mocha, said. "He said he's had them once before."

Julie glanced at Tom, who shook his head and frowned just enough to convey his surprise at the information.

"You didn't know?" the doctor asked, opening a door and motioning them into an empty office.

"No," Julie admitted. Her stomach churned. She was unsure whether it was from her worries about Pete or from the drugs she was taking. In either case, she had to find out what was wrong with Pete. "Diagnosis?"

"We'll have to run some tests," the doctor began. His words were slow and chosen with care, as one does who deals with people in high-stress situations when giving and receiving precise information can be strewn with misunderstanding—deadly misunderstandings.

"I'm a neurosurgeon on staff at Mount Hermon," Julie said. Being a doctor had its advantages and one of them was getting more information out of other doctors than most people did, or could. "What do you suspect and which tests are you ordering?"

The doctor sniffed, rubbed his clean-shaven chin with his long fingers and said, glancing at Tom and then Christy, "Steroid use."

"Impossible," Julie said shaking her head.

"He has many of the symptoms," the doctor said, and then, seeing Julie's stern face, added, "it could be something else." He sounded as if he would be shocked if it wasn't steroids.

"It must be something else," Julie insisted.

"Why do you think he's using steroids?" Tom asked, his brow wrinkled with concern.

"Acne, hair loss, decreased sex drive, enlarged jaw and heart palpitations."

"Decreased sex drive?" Julie asked, shocked.

The doctor nodded.

"How....I don't....what?" Julie struggled to form a question.

"Self report," the doctor said. Pete was underage, so the doctor could tell Pete's parents about his condition. "In any case, he's on an IV drip and his heart palpitations have ceased. I'd like to keep him here a little longer to make sure he's stable and then you can take him home. He needs to see a cardiologist though, soon."

Julie closed her eyes and sighed with relief as the tension eased from her shoulders and neck. The nightmare was over—or at least it was receding back into the night.

"Get back to writing," her father told her.

Julie's eyes flicked wide open and darted around the tiny office. "What?" It had been her father's voice, clear and distinct, yet he was nowhere to be seen. She trembled, afraid and uncertain.

"I recommend a blood test," the doctor said. Hadn't he heard her father?

Concentrating on what the doctor had said, Julie said, "We'll have our internist do it."

"A writer writes," her father told her. Julie gritted her teeth. He was not here. He could not be here. He was in Carlsbad.

The ER doctor nodded, but glanced at Tom with a meaningful look before stepping out of the room to see his next patient.

"You need to finish your novel now," her father admonished Julie. She told herself her father was not present, regardless of how real his voice sounded. It was an auditory hallucination from the drugs she was taking. The drugs increased creativity and also increased misfires in the brain, causing hallucinations of the olfactory, visual and now auditory kind. Her father was not present.

"Steroids?" Tom said, half a question, half an appalled statement.

"Of course not," Julie snapped.

"Are you certain? You mentioned his sudden rage before."

"I'm a doctor. You don't think I'd notice if my son was taking steroids?"

"You're also his mother," Tom said, his voice soothing.

Julie glared at Tom. "I can look after my son."

"Our son."

"I better go see if he's alright."

"You have to write to get published."

In her mind, Julie told her father to shut up as she strode across the hall to see Pete.

"The various committees have met," the Chair of Neurosurgery, Andrew Baxter began without preamble in his office, "and have made their decision."

Julie braced herself. With Pete recovered from his Friday night ordeal, Monday morning found her about to be told whether she would keep her job at Mount Hermon. She sat across from Baxter in the most respectable outfit she owned; a simple black knee-length skirt and white blouse—the outfit her father liked so much. Even with the drugs she was taking to counteract the side effects of the clinical trial drugs, she still suffered. The side effects were far worse when she was under stress, and she was under stress. Her head ached, her stomach churned and her blood pressure, which she had checked that morning, had hit dangerous highs. At least she had suffered no hallucinations this morning.

"Unanimous, I should tell you." Baxter looked across his desk, waited a moment, and said, "The decision is that you are welcome to resume your position at Mount Hermon with all the rights and privileges of an attending faculty member."

Julie's spirit soared. She had her life back.

"Under one condition."

"One condition?" Julie trembled as her spirit froze and fear flooded her body.

"A drug test."

The meaning of those three little words sank into Julie's brain, the implications rippling out in ever-larger waves of repercussions until they formed a tidal wave of terror. "I don't," she began.

"There's no room for negotiation," Baxter said, raising his hand to stop her in mid-sentence. "It's simple. If you want your position back, you submit to a drug test today, and then weekly until the Chief of Staff is satisfied that you are no longer taking any of the drugs from your clinical trial."

"Why should that matter?"

"Why should it matter?" Baxter demanded, dumbfounded by the question. "Those drugs are not approved by the FDA or by anyone else for use in combination, let alone for someone with no medical condition or disease."

"They increase creativity."

"No research supports your unfounded belief that they do anything other than induce a range of negative side effects, including increasing the risk of TIAs and strokes. If you take them, it makes me, the committees and the Chief of Staff seriously question your decision-making ability and judgment."

"The drugs are not illegal."

"Writing prescriptions for yourself is against the rules of the state medical board."

"Everyone does it."

"For gingivitis and flu; not for taking drugs from a clinical trial that's been terminated because a patient died."

"He was geriatric and had Alzheimer's. I'm young and healthy. The risks are insignificant."

"You don't know what the risks are. No one's ever tested that drug combination."

"I have some data—"

"A few months' worth; nothing to risk your life on."

Julie fell silent. Baxter was right, at least to the extent that she didn't know the risks.

"I don't see a problem," Baxter said, the voice of calm reason. Their eyes met. "You have discontinued taking them, haven't you?"

It should not have happened. In his locker, Pete kept a plastic tube full of clean urine: it contained no drugs, anabolic steroids, anti-histamine or anything else the state High School Athletic Commission deemed illegal. Mike Lowe, his steroid connection, had supplied the clean urine for $100 a month. Pete would have just asked a friend to supply it, but he didn't want anyone else to know he was using. Weekly Mike supplied a new tube. From his research on the Internet, Mike was fairly certain the urine degraded and after a week a lab might be able to tell it wasn't fresh. The nurse collecting the samples sometimes checked their temperature by issuing vials with temperature strips on them. For that reason Mike stressed that Pete should tape the tube to the inside of his thigh for at least 10 minutes before using it for a drug test so the urine would be the right temperature. It was, he told Pete, a failsafe system; failsafe except for Pete's mom.

"One-thirty-five over eighty-eight," she proclaimed that morning as she undid the blood pressure cuff on his arm. Intent on devouring his breakfast, Pete paid scant attention to her during this now daily morning ritual. "A little high."

"I'm in a rush," Pete said. He had overslept after a restless night. The Rogaine appeared to be working, but it made his scalp itchy to the point where he couldn't sleep. Luckily, his mom didn't know about the Rogaine.

"You're heart's running a little fast, too," she said, putting her stethoscope back in one of the pockets of her lab coat, where it hung in the front hall closet. "Maybe you should skip practice this morning."

"I'm fine, Mom." He finished eating and rushed with his dishes into the kitchen to put them in the dishwasher with a clatter.

"I'll call the coach and tell him you'll miss practice today," his mom said with a note of finality, which he hated. He wasn't a kid anymore.

"Mom," Pete whined. "The cardiologist said I was fine." His mom had used her clout, or what was left of it, to get him in to see one of the top cardiologists at Mount Hermon the Tuesday after his ER visit.

"Just for today."

"If I miss practice, Jayden and Cain will get to play Friday, not me."

"You can practice tomorrow."

"I need to practice, Mom, today."

"Calm down, Pete. Just this one morning, for me, alright? I'm worried about you. You had heart palpitations. It's serious, Pete."

"I'm going," Pete said, grabbing his bag out of the hall closet as his anger mounted.

"No, you're not. I'm calling the coach."

"I'm fine and I'm going."

"Pete, stop right now," his mom yelled.

Ignoring his mother, Pete, rushed out the front door.

When he arrived at school, Pete was about to hurry into the locker room when one of the assistant coaches on his way out to the field spotted him and yelled, "Tomlinson, what are you doing here?"

"Practicing," Pete yelled back as if it was a stupid question.

"No way," the assistant said, shaking his sun-tanned head. "I just spoke with your mom. She said you're sick and you'd be missing practice today."

"I'm fine, coach."

"Your mom says you aren't."

"I am."

"You're mom says you aren't, you aren't. She's the voice of God on this one."

Pete swore and thumped the locker room door with his fist.

"Everyone gets sick, Tomlinson. Take it easy."

Pete spun on his heel to stalk off, but before he took three strides, the coach called out, "Wait, Tomlinson. I almost forgot. You've been selected. Come on. The others are already with the nurse."

Pete froze. This could not be happening. When routine drug tests were scheduled, everyone knew beforehand that the nurse from the commission was on campus. It was different if someone had already failed a test; in those cases it was well nigh impossible to cheat. But for the routine tests, once he heard that the nurse was on campus, Pete taped the urine-sample tube to his thigh. Then he was ready if he was one of the players randomly selected for testing as the team trouped from the locker room out to the practice fields. Thus far, he hadn't been selected. His luck had run out at the worst possible time and it was all his mom's fault. If she hadn't delayed him and kept him out of practice, he would have been ready for the test, urine tube taped to his leg.

"Just let me drop my bag off in the locker room," Pete said, pushing the door open, the pungent odor of the locker room assaulting his nostrils.

"No way. Once you've been told, I have to stay with you until I deliver you to the nurse. Come on, I've got to get out to the field."

Rage coursed through Pete's body, locking his jaw into place and filling him with anger. Every muscle in his body tensed, every nerve taut. It was all her fault. He slammed a fist into the door with a resounding thump that echoed down the hall.

"That's enough, Tomlinson, come on," the coach ordered, his face set in a stern, commanding glare. "Now!"

Julie loaded her bulging files of rejection letters from agents, publishers and literary journals into a white cardboard box and slapped on the lid. She surveyed her office at Mount Hermon, now a cluster of boxes, bare shelves and an empty desk. Was she was out of her mind? She was in disgrace. Her colleagues who had heard what had happened must think she was crazy. Her brain screamed at her that she had to stop taking the drugs, take the drug test and keep her job at Mount Hermon. Her heart said otherwise. The drugs were opening the gate to a path that would lead to writing a great novel and becoming a novelist. She had to write.

"I hear via my assistant's gossip circuit that you're leaving us," thrice-divorced neurosurgeon Rick Severn said as he strolled into her office. Glancing around, he added, "I liked your office the way you had it: far more lived in."

Julie smiled despite herself, and said, "You heard right."

"Such a shame; I had high hopes for us. I thought we had something, or at least something that might become something." Hands in his pants' pockets, he looked sad and full of loss.

"I must have missed something," Julie said, suppressing a smile despite her worries.

"Women often do," Severn said. "All that crap about women being the more emotionally sensitive sex is just plain wrong. Men know what's going on; well, at least when love and sex are involved."

"Well, at least with the later."

"I thought, given time and maybe a few lunches—"

"With or without pharma reps?"

Severn gave her a pained looked. "A few lunches, getting to know each other a little better, and we might have had some fun together. Maybe even something long term."

"My word, Dr. Severn, are you proposing marriage?" Julie asked with a coquettish look, as she tried to keep from laughing.

"Of course not. Three alimony payments is quite enough for any man."

"So what then?"

"Oh, maybe some fun between the sheets."

"I think I could have you up on sexual harassment charges."

"I doubt it. I'm on that committee, too." He gave an exaggerated, dramatic sigh and, taking a wad of papers from his pocket, reached out to hand them to Julie. "I've collected these over the past few months. Thought you could use them to ease the strain."

Julie frowned as she reached for them. "What are they?"

"Coupons for free meals at various and sundry fine restaurants in the area. The various people I've dined with have been more than kind in seeing that I never lack for a free meal, contrary to the old saw that such a thing is merely a myth."

Julie withdrew her empty hand. "Thanks, but I think I'll pass."

Severn's voice became serious, "Julie, my dear, times could become rather financially tough before you find another position." He glanced at the open door, listened a moment and, hearing nothing, added in a whisper, "Baxter is spreading it around that you are, shall we say, far from reliable, possibly even as I heard it put on the BBC America the other night, a nutter. I think he's hurt that you let him down or, more likely, that you made him look bad by doing such a thing under his command. Please, take the coupons."

"I'll be fine, but thanks, Rick."

He still held out the wad of coupons.

"Truly, I'll be fine."

After a long moment, he nodded, stuffed the coupons back in his pleated-pant's pocket and, rocking back on his heels, asked, "I suppose the offer of some frolicking fun times between the sheets is also an unreasonable and steadfast no?"

Touched, Julie smiled. "Steadfast, but not unreasonable; reluctant."

He smiled with mock fortitude, bid her farewell and sauntered out the door and down the hall.

Julie picked up her bag and walked over to Sandy's cubicle. "Thank you for all the support over the years."

"It's been a pleasure, well, most of it," she said with a broad smile. Sandy hugged Julie.

As they hugged, Julie whispered, "Whatever you've heard—"

"Doesn't change the fact that you were great to work for," Sandy interrupted. "If you ever need another assistant, give me a call."

They stared at each other for a long moment before the middle-aged Sandy asked in a maternal tone, "I know this may be out of line and none of my business and I promised myself I wouldn't ask, but why in the name of Heaven didn't you just take the drug test?"

"I couldn't."

They stared at each other and Julie was relieved that Sandy knew her well enough not to ask again.

Julie's plan for a quick exit was foiled at every step by nurses, management assistants, researchers and physicians who wished her well, hugged her and said goodbye. It took her 50 minutes to make it out the institute's front door, having explained for the twentieth time that she planned to take some time off before seeing what opportunities were out there. She, and everyone she told, knew this was code for her having nothing lined up.

In the restroom, Pete nodded at the male nurse lounging against the sinks as he handed Pete a clear vial. It had a temperature strip, not that it mattered, not today. Pete passed six open stall doors and spotted teammates, including Cain and the sophomore safety, Manny Ortiz, who looked excited to be involved in his first drug test. Their bags, jackets and personal belongings were outside, but due to a state ruling that required they be given "absolute privacy" for the actual provision of their sample, the stall doors would be closed when they gave their sample.

Pete found an empty stall at the end. The water in the toilet was blue to ensure that no one could dilute their sample in an attempt to fool the testing. Glancing back, he realized it would have been so easy. He could hear the nurse walking down the row of stalls to check on each of them just before and after they provided their sample. Timing when to use the clean sample, if he had it, would have been as easy as tackling a five-year-old girl.

Pete used his own urine to fill the sample vial. Head down, shoulders slumped, he handed it in, praying the delivery service would lose it, a lab tech would drop it or lightening would strike the lab and burn it to the ground before the test was run—anything to save him and his NFL future.

As Pete left the restroom, Cain strode past him. Glancing back and seeing only Pete in the hall lined with athletic trophy cases, Cain reached down the inside of his tight football pants and tore out a flexible, plastic hose about eight inches long. Two pieces of white surgical tape dangled from it. Cain tossed the tube into a trashcan, cast a triumphant smirk back at Pete and slammed open the doors to trot out to the practice fields.

Choose a job you love and
you'll never have to work a day in your life.

—Confucius

Julie sat at her desk at home searching for a job on the Internet. She found some tantalizing positions for a neurosurgeon with clinical and research expertise at Johns Hopkins, the University of South Carolina, the University of Nevada, Reno, the Mayo Clinic, the University of New Brunswick in Canada, and at the University of Hawaii Medical Center. She thought she could sweet talk a couple of carefully selected colleagues into writing her letters of recommendation that would gloss over the reason she had abruptly left Mount Hermon. She could claim she was just looking for a change. Hawaii would be a nice change. Maybe Reno would take a gamble on her. Yet, even as her mind wandered down happy paths of relocating to Hawaii for the climate or Mayo or Hopkins for the prestige, one major problem turned all of the paths into abrupt dead ends: Pete.

In his final year in high school, Pete could not move. They could not move, at least until June—eight months away. It might take that long to find a new position, but Julie's savings couldn't cover their bills for eight months without a paycheck. Abruptly going from earning in the mid-six figures to zero meant that her savings were decreasing at an alarming rate even as she tried to cut costs with a ruthless eye. Regardless of any reductions in spending, her largest bills could not be cut. Her father's nursing home cost $75,000 a year, which Julie had offered to cover when her job appeared secure. If she had not, her parents would have run out of money years ago. Her mortgage ran to $7,500 a month. With the recent downturn in the housing market, she had little equity in her home and even if she did, no bank would allow her to refinance to take out any equity if she was unemployed. During the divorce, Julie had fought hard to keep the house, so Pete wouldn't have to move on top of having his parents split up. Unluckily, she had bought out Tom at the top of the market. Tom also had been awarded reimbursement alimony: alimony awarded to someone who supports their spouse while they go to school only to have the marriage end soon after the spouse starts making money as a doctor or lawyer. It is awarded to wives who earn Ph.T's: Put Him Through, but in Julie's case it was awarded to Tom, since he supported her while she went to medical school. She had been paying Tom 30 percent of her income until recently, when Tom finally married Christy after what to Julie seemed an endless courtship. Julie was still paying off the last of her student loans, which had reached $175,000 by the time she graduated medical school. All of it made what appeared to be a handsome salary into one that barely covered her bills.

Now with no income she would run out of money in about six months. She loathed the idea of moving her father to a cheaper nursing home or selling the house to downsize to a condo and moving Pete, but if she didn't find a job soon, she might have to consider doing both.

She regretted not saving more money before but the divorce, Pete, her father, college funds for her neices, and so many other things had made demands on her purse that had all seemed reasonable at the time. Now she realized that she had been far too generous. She had always thought she could save more for herself later.

For an instant she considered having Pete live with Tom so she could try to find a job in another city, but the thought of losing her son was unthinkable. She would lose him the following fall when he went away to college, but she still harbored an unspoken dream that he would choose USC or UCLA. That way he could stay at home four more precious years. Then, she thought with a smile, he could do graduate work at either school and he might be home another five or six years, if he did a doctorate. She didn't want to lose him, not yet, not so soon.

Sighing, she accepted the reality that she had to find a position in Los Angeles. She knew before she even looked on various websites that positions for neurosurgeons were rare, let alone if you limited your search to one city, no matter how large. The United States had about 3,600 neurosurgeons and there were only 7,400 in the world; a rarified group. People who worked outside medicine probably believed that any neurosurgeon, being such a rare commodity, would be able to secure a job anywhere they wanted. The reality was that only a relative few hospitals could afford a neurosurgery program. Neurosurgeons required specialized diagnostic and OR equipment, nurses, staff, malpractice insurance, which could run $200,000 a year for each neurosurgeon, and, in many cases, lab space. Neurosurgery could generate significant income for a hospital, but a neurosurgical program was costly to establish, especially since more than one neurosurgeon was required for a viable program. With such requirements, it was no surprise that there were only about 30 or 40 such programs in all of California. Job openings were rare.

After an hour, Julie found no positions in LA County. The closest position was in San Diego, which might have been doable but it was for a spine specialist. She could do spine, but since her residency she had specialized in the OR on pituitary and vascular conditions: arteriovenous malformations, aneurysms and strokes. If she applied, they would be far more likely to hire a spine specialist.

Looking out the window, she wondered what Alan was doing. Had he read her chapters? What did he think? Did he think her mad? Probably.

Grabbing a cup of coffee and pushing thoughts of Alan from her mind, she decided that she had better keep looking instead of working on her novel. She searched for other possible positions in Los Angeles. Maybe she could find employment as a general practitioner, researcher or physician for a sports team or something. It would be difficult to convince someone that a neurosurgeon was qualified, let alone wanted a non-neurosurgical position, but she had to try. Her savings were vanishing at an alarming rate. She had to find a job.

Some people think football is a matter of life and death. I assure you, it's much more serious than that.

—Bill Shankly, Scottish football [soccer] player and manager, 1913-1981

"Your son failed a drug test." It was Coach Paukenan on the phone.

In her home office, Julie stopped scanning a list of medical job openings on her computer. "What drugs were found?"

"Anabolic steroids."

"There must be some mistake." Even as she said it she knew everyone who failed such a test said the same thing, and all their mothers said it too.

"The lab runs the test twice to be certain. Both came back positive. They have a 99.99 percent accuracy rate. That's why the state athletic commission uses them."

"They sound rigorous," Julie admitted, although she was already familiar with how much care labs devoted to conducting such tests.

"Are there any medications he is on that might account for a false positive?"

"None." Julie took a deep breath and asked, "What happens now?"

"Pete is suspended for a week. Then we'll retest him. If he passes, he'll be tested weekly for the rest of the season. If he fails the second test, a third test will be given one week later."

"If he fails that test?"

"He's off the team for the remainder of his time in high school."

Julie closed her eyes, exhaled and said a silent prayer that this was not happening. "What did he say?"

"In such cases, we inform the parents first. It's up to them how they want to communicate it to the student-athlete."

Julie hung up and the phone rang. It was Pete's father, Tom, who demanded, "What the hell's going on with Pete?"

"Don't shout at me."

"I get a call from his coach saying he failed a drug test; steroids. Did you know?" Tom asked, his voice betraying that he believed she must have known.

"Of course I didn't know. I would never let him do that."

"The doctor at the ER said he might be using steroids. Didn't that give you a hint? I thought he might be, but I believed you were better qualified to notice such things. Given all his symptons—"

"My God, Tom, every teenager has acne and has mood swings," Julie said, her voice rising in anger. "I didn't think Pete would do such a stupid thing. He's a good kid."

"Apparently not."

"He made a mistake. We'll handle it." Then, realizing what she had said might be misinterpreted, she added, "Pete and I will take care of it." She had divorced Tom in part because he could never let her run her own life. The last thing she wanted was Tom meddling in her and Pete's life any more than was absolutely necessary.

"What are we going to do?" Tom asked, ignoring Julie's clarification of who would handle the problem.

"I," Julie said, emphasizing the word, "will talk to Pete. He will stop using steroids."

"Agreed. Maybe he should come live with me for a while."

"No," Julie spat back, appalled at the idea.

"It's just a thought," Tom said, sounding more conciliatory. "I know football."

"I know my son."

"He just might be too much for you to handle right now. He's a young man now."

"I can handle him."

"Apparently not, Julie. He's on steroids and I hear you've been fired from Mount Hermon." Tom paused, as if deciding whether to delve further into the matter. "Why?"

"I'll take care of my son. I always have and I will continue to do so." Julie hung up.

*In the very books in which philosophers bid us
scorn fame, they inscribe their names.*

—Cicero

As soon as Julie walked into Pete's room late that afternoon, any doubt she harbored about her son using steroids vanished. As he sat in his treasured Bears jersey at his desk reading a battered, graffiti-marred textbook, she saw that the hair at the top of his head was thinner, showing a glimpse of sun-reddened skin beneath. When he turned, she could not help but notice the acne alongside his nostrils and across his forehead, as well as an irregular pattern of pockmarks at various stages of healing that dotted his once-pristine face. She realized that his chin had enlarged over the past few months, as had his entire body. No amount of weight training and eating right could naturally produce such muscle mass in so short a time. Looking at him with clear eyes for the first time in months, she realized he was a classic case of steroid use. Seeing him every day, she had missed the gradual changes in him. The fear of what the steroids could have done to his body made her sick. She swallowed hard and forced herself to regain control.

"You're using steroids," she said without preamble.

He frowned. "No, I'm not." The words came fast as if he was repeating a mantra he had practiced a thousand times before, if not in reality, at least in his mind for just such a moment. He didn't even look surprised.

"Don't bother, Pete." She slumped on his bed. "Coach called with the results of your drug test."

"It's a mistake."

"No," Julie said, keeping her voice even and calm, "it's not."

"It must be."

"No," she said, her voice rising. "Give me some credit, Pete. I know how careful labs are with testing, especially drug testing, so they can be certain." She met his stare and, after a moment, his gaze fell to the floor. "You have to stop."

"I'm not taking…"

"Stop it, Pete!" Julie yelled. "That's enough. I'm not that stupid."

A look of surprise on his face, Pete turned back to his textbook. After a few moments, he turned his gaze to meet her eyes again and said, "I'll lose my spot on the team."

"You're already off the team for a week or longer until you can pass another drug test."

"I'll pass it, no problem."

"The steroids will still be in your system."

"I'll pass."

"They aren't going to let you use someone else's urine, dilute yours with a massive intake of water or try to fool the test with some other half-baked scheme. They know you've been using. They'll know if you've quit."

"The state requires that my privacy be ensured while I give my sample."

"They aren't going to let you take anything in with you when you provide the sample. They'll have you strip down to your undershorts." Julie sighed and shook her head. "The test is beside the point. The point is I don't want you taking steroids. You aren't taking steroids. They damage your body. They're serious, Pete."

"They're not illegal."

"They are without a prescription, and high school athletes are not allowed to take them."

"No one gets arrested for taking steroids."

"I'm not having this argument, Pete. It doesn't matter if society says they're illegal or not, or if they arrest people for steroid use or not. I don't want you taking them."

"If I stop using, I'll lose my linebacking spot."

"Maybe you can play tight end."

"I want to be a linebacker, and if I don't take steroids, coach will use Jayden and Cain as his linebackers and tight ends."

"You're a good tight end."

"I'm getting tackled by safeties for God's sake."

"You may get cut, but even if you do, it's not worth your health or your life."

"I won't have a life without football."

"Of course you will."

"I've played football my whole life. Without it, I'll have nothing."

"You'll have a future, a career doing something, you'll have me, your dad, friends, Amanda—"

"We broke up."

Surprised, Julie stopped short. "I'm sorry to hear that." She wondered what other secrets he was holding close to his heart besides steroids and losing a girlfriend, but she knew this was not the time to ask. "I hope you were….careful when you were with her."

"Of course," Pete said with a dismissive wave of his hand. He stood and stalked across the room to the window, where he stared out into the night. He had never liked closing his blinds. He liked looking out at the stars, at least the few that could be seen in light-polluted LA. "Everyone on the team uses them. I can't compete if I don't."

His voice was low and Julie strained to hear him. She was uncertain whether it was a justification, an explanation or just a statement to break the tense silence that buzzed between them.

"I don't care if the entire country is using them," Julie said. "You aren't."

"If I don't, I'm off the team. I tried all winter and spring to add muscle without them and gained a couple of pounds. It was useless."

"Then you're off the team, period. No discussion, no debate. That's final."

He turned to face her. His body was tense, his face a picture of anger, bordering on rage. His voice rose as he said, "Football's the most important thing in my life. It's all I care about, all I am. I want to play college ball and then in the pros."

"The steroids will kill you," Julie said, standing to face him.

"If I drop dead the day after I retire from the NFL, I'll have had a good life."

"You could drop dead tomorrow or, worse, a stroke could incapacitate you so that you can't even hold a football."

"You just don't understand," Pete screamed.

"You will stop taking steroids," Julie ordered, tired of the pointless argument. The end was preordained: Pete would stop taking steroids.

"No!" he screamed, his red, anger-filled face inches from her face.

"Pete, never yell at me like that!"

"I'm going to do whatever it takes to play football!"

"Not under my roof!"

"Then I'll go live with Dad."

"He won't let you take steroids either."

"Then I'll move out on my own."

He brushed by her to leave, but she grabbed his muscular arm. In an instant he had grabbed her wrist and, spinning her around, slammed her into the wall. A glass-covered, autographed photograph of Mike Singletary fell and clattered to the floor, its glob of earthquake putty stuck uselessly to the frame. As she hit the wall, Julie felt her wrist snap. A wave of pain followed by nausea swept over her, clouding her vision of her enraged son. She groaned and, falling to her knees, cradled her snapped right wrist with her left hand.

"Pete," Julie gasped as he stalked out his bedroom door. Her voice a mixture of anguish, pain and sorrow, she called again, "Pete."

Life isn't long enough for love and art.

—Somerset Maugham,
The Moon and Sixpence, 1919

"We'll have to go in and align the bones," Dr. Short explained to Julie. He was one of the top orthopaedic surgeons in the country and was an attending at Mount Hermon. "Probably next week, after the inflammation subsides."

"Will I be able to operate again?" Julie asked from the bed in the ER cubicle. Pete stood, head down, shoulders slumped, as far to the side of the cubicle as he could be without standing behind the white curtain that separated it from the next cubicle.

"With intensive rehab, you should regain complete range of motion and strength in the wrist and fingers," Short said with a reassuring smile. "There might be a minor deficit, but you won't notice it. You should be able to operate with as much precision as you did before. Besides, I thought all you neurosurgeons used robots to assist you now anyways."

"Only on the tricky procedures."

"Especially the ones the marketing types mention?" Short asked with a knowing grin.

Julie nodded, relieved that her wrist and hand would be alright. She looked down at the cast that now covered her arm from the first digit of her fingers to her shoulder. It felt as if it weighed 60 pounds. She wondered if she would be able to fit through doorways and shuddered at the thought of trying to sleep, eat or bathe with the white monstrosity encasing her arm.

"Come to see me about the middle of next week," Short said. He picked up Julie's medical file from off a metal table and said, "The X-rays showed osteoporosis. You're pretty young to have it." Short's brown eyes narrowed, waiting for more information from his patient.

"It's common in my family," Julie said, swinging her legs off the examination table to go home.

"Are you taking something for it?"

"Yes."

Short tapped the file on his thigh.

Julie added, "A bisphosphonate."

"I also noticed your blood pressure is a little high and your heart rate is elevated."

Julie looked at him with a look of warning.

After a quick glance at Pete, Short ignored the warning and plunged ahead. "Your blood test showed elevated liver enzyme levels, as well as a brew of drugs I'd hesitate to prescribe to anyone in combination. Your EKG showed intermittent heart palpitations. I'd recommend a visit to a cardiologist, and stopping the drugs you're taking. I assume they're the drug combination from your clinical trial?"

Hospitals, even one like Mount Hermon with 8,000 employees and more than 2,000 physicians, were little villages with rumors spreading faster than any infectious disease.

"I know what I'm doing," Julie said.

Short glanced over at Pete again. The orthopaedic surgeon straightened, slapped the file against his thigh, and sniffed. "I hope so, Dr. Stein, I truly hope so," he said, assuming a formal tone. "I heard one of your trial patients died."

"I'm aware of that."

Short looked as if he was debating whether to continue the conversation. He decided against it. Julie accepted a prescription for when the pain-killing shot she had received wore off, and in a curt tone thanked Short.

"I'll order a wheelchair and you can go," Short said, his voice cold and businesslike.

"I don't need a wheelchair," Julie said, brooking no disagreement. She rose, getting the feel of the enormous cast. It seemed overkill for a broken wrist, but it was necessary to keep the wrist and its eight carpal bones and four joints immobile. Even so, as she stood, something shifted, causing a pain as if someone had stabbed her in the wrist. She winced and leaned against the bed, almost falling.

"You alright?" Pete asked, rushing toward her.

For the first time in her life, Julie felt fear when she saw him coming.

"I'm fine," she gasped as the sharp pain passed as suddenly as it had struck. Regardless of what he had done, she told herself, she should never be afraid of her son.

As she led Pete along a white corridor toward the entrance, he said, "I'm sorry, Mom." He looked down and his shoulders slumped in dejection.

"I know. You don't have to keep saying it." He had said he was sorry repeatedly as he had rushed her to the hospital as fast as he could while breaking only a half-dozen traffic laws. Julie had vetoed an ambulance. Her wrist was broken and an extra couple of minutes driving to the hospital would make little difference.

Pete fell silent as they plodded across the deserted parking structure toward his car. It was 2:15 a.m.

"What was he talking about the clinical trial for?" Pete asked. "I thought it was cancelled."

"It was." It still sometimes threw Julie when Pete, her baby boy, acted like an adult, listening to conversations that just a few years before he would have ignored or, if he listened, he wouldn't have understood.

"Why are you taking drugs from the trial? You don't have Alzheimer's, do you?"

Julie stopped, realizing what she thought Pete was thinking. "No, Pete, I do not have Alzheimer's."

He pursed his lips and said, his voice low, "I'm sorry, Mom. I don't know what came over me. I just lost it."

She put her good arm around him, wincing as the movement sent a burning pain down her injured arm. "I know it was the steroids, not you, Pete. I know you'd never hurt me on purpose."

Pete nodded, his head still down.

She got up on her toes and kissed his cheek.

"That's why you have to stop taking steroids," she said as they approached his BMW. "Not only the 'roid rage, but the heart palpitations, the acne, the hair loss and, far more seriously, the potential damage to your liver, kidneys, heart and body, including your sexual function."

Even in the semi-darkness of the parking structure at night, Pete looked away at the mention of sex.

Julie said, "Nothing is as important as your health."

They reached the car. Pete helped her with great gentleness and care into the passenger seat of his BMW. He slid in behind the wheel.

"If you don't have Alzheimer's, why are you taking the drugs from your clinical trial?" He sat, left hand on the wheel, his right on the key in the ignition. "I thought they didn't work."

"They do," Julie spat back.

Pete noted her tone and glanced at her.

"At least they appear to," she added in a more even tone. "Memory, cognitive function and creativity all improved."

"Then why'd they stop the trial?"

"We should go, Pete. It's late."

"You said someone died?"

"My arm's hurting and I'd like to fill the prescription so I can take some pain meds before I go to bed, assuming I can get any sleep with this thing." She gestured with her chin down at the white cast, which was wrapped in blue, stretchy fabric.

"Someone died?"

Julie sighed. She was tired, hurting and this was the last time or place she wanted to discuss her study, let alone with Pete. She had lost her job and a potential boyfriend, her son was on steroids, and now she had a broken wrist. Seeing that Pete was not going to abandon this line of questioning, she said in a bored tone as if she was reciting a government report, "A patient in the trial had a stroke and died. When that happens, a study is evaluated and, in this case, a board of researchers and physicians decided to suspend the trial."

"Why are you taking drugs that killed somebody?"

Julie's first thought was to tell him it was none of his business, but in looking over at him, she saw not a boy who could be lied to or manipulated into a version of reality she wanted him to believe, but a young man with a quick mind. He was the son of a neurosurgeon and, as much as she hated to admit it, Tom, his father, was far from stupid. Tom was a successful businessman and had a mind that was as quick as any neurosurgeon. If Tom had been stupid, she never would have married him. Because of his quick mind, Pete was far from easy to lie to, and the perseverance that had allowed Julie to become a neurosurgeon, complete challenging, multi-year research studies and continue writing fiction with no success for years, was also ingrained in him. He would not drop this topic until he received a satisfactory answer.

She scrunched her eyes shut for a moment, wishing she could go to sleep or even just find a position in which the mammoth cast felt comfortable, but she knew that neither was to be achieved anytime soon, especially if she didn't answer Pete's questions.

She said, "The drugs appear to increase creativity."

"So?"

"Creativity such as—"

"To write novels," Pete finished her sentence. "But you might die from a stroke?"

"The patient in my study who died was far older than I am and had many pre-existing health conditions, which I do not have."

"But you could die?"

"As I said, he was in his late sixties, had several life-threatening health conditions—"

"You could die."

Julie looked out over the city from the parking structure. The hills of Ladera Heights and Baldwin Hills across the valley that cradled Los Angeles rose in the distance as a patchwork of lights in the semi-darkness of the megalopolis.

She said, "Yes."

"You can't…Why…I don't understand."

"I've been trying to be a writer since I was born," Julie said, still looking out over the sleeping city as she tried to answer the jumble of questions embodied in her son's half-question. "I've never had much success writing fiction. I've given up a dozen times, but I can't. It's a part of me; it's in my blood. I have to be a writer. The drug combination from the trial has made it far easier to write and to write well. The agent who called loved the sample chapters I sent him and a publisher wants to publish my novel. That would never have happened without the drugs."

"It would have."

"It hadn't in more than 20 years of trying."

"But you could die."

Julie looked over at her son. "I love writing. Neurosurgery is great and I like it, even love it at times, but it's nowhere close to writing. On a scale of 1 to 10, neurosurgery is a 10; writing is a thousand."

"Like me and football?"

"Not at all like you and football," Julie exclaimed, shocked and furious at the comparison.

"How's it different?" Pete asked, his voice calm.

"They're completely different," Julie said, fighting to return her voice to a normal level to match Pete's reasonable tone.

"You want to be a writer. I want to be a football player. We both took drugs to do it."

"You can't compare steroids to the drugs in my study," Julie said, appalled at the comparison.

"They can both kill you."

Julie glared out the side window, not wanting Pete to see her anger. Why couldn't they just go home? It was so late and she was exhausted. Taking a deep breath and turning back to her son, she said, "I'm an adult. I can make decisions like this. You're still a kid."

"I'm not."

"I'm not saying it to put you down, but you are a kid. You don't have the experience and knowledge older people have. You don't realize—"

"I realize you could die."

"I'm not going to die," Julie said, her exasperation increasing. "I'm monitoring my condition and I'm doing fine."

"Were you monitoring the patients in your study?"

Julie looked at her son, wishing he was still the little boy she could deceive with white lies.

"I have to do this, Pete."

"I have to take steroids so I can keep playing football." He said it evenly, but with a flood of emotion behind the simple words. "To make the team, let alone the first string, even in high school, you have to be so good, so fast, so strong. You can't do it anymore without steroids. Jayden and Cain use them, and so does every running back I have to stop. I got run over in a few games last year and this year it would have been far worse if I hadn't bulked up."

"If you hadn't taken steroids."

"Yes, I took steroids."

"You cheated."

"Is it cheating if everyone does it?"

Julie didn't know how to answer that.

Pete said, "Home run hitters in baseball, Olympic track stars, cyclists and football players all take steroids. The better ones even end up in the Hall of Fame. How can it be wrong?"

"Sometimes society is wrong," Julie said. "Look, it's not the same, and I don't want to have this argument." She knew how their last argument had ended, even though she told herself Pete would never hurt her again.

"Why is it different?" His voice was calm and even. Why couldn't he just throw a tantrum and lose his temper? It would obviate any need for her to defend her position with reason and logic, let alone to try to explain.

Julie sighed. "Our age, to start with."

"So it's alright for you to risk your life, but not me?"

"You have so much of your life ahead of you. Football can only be a part of your life for a few short years. You told me once that the average career of a football player in the pros is what? Three years? Four?"

"It's not like you don't have a long life ahead of you. You could live another 50 years."

"Football just isn't that important."

"It is. If it wasn't, why does a section of the newspaper and entire websites cover sports? Why are whole magazines devoted to football? Millions of people know the names of pros. Why do they pay players millions a year? Way more than you make as a neurosurgeon. You save lives and they play a game, but they get paid millions and little kids write for their autographs. Does anyone want your autograph?"

"It's football. It's just a game. It's not art or literature."

"Who cares about art or books? How popular are writers compared to athletes? At school they put up the pictures of all the football players who made All State."

"They post pictures of the Merit Scholars, too."

"In the basement of the science wing. They're tiny and they aren't even framed." The disdain was clear in Pete's voice. "Millions of people watch football on television."

"I'm sure ten times more people attend a play, see a movie, go to an art gallery or buy a novel in a given year than ever attend a football game."

"Sports are huge on TV. No one watches art on television."

"There are TV shows on art, plays and adaptations of novels on television, and all movies and television shows are a form of art. Besides, in a hundred years, no one will remember any football players' names. I don't know the names of any wrestlers, boxers or athletes from ancient Greece, Rome or Elizabethan England, but everyone's heard of Sophocles and Euripides, Cicero and Seneca, Thomas Marlowe and Shakespeare."

"I've never heard of them," Pete spat back, "except Shake-speare."

"Then you should pay more attention in English class."

They fell silent.

"'If a writer has to rob his mother, he will not hesitate; the 'Ode on a Grecian Urn' is worth any number of old ladies.'" Julie mumbled.

"What?"

"Just a novelist, William Faulkner, talking about devotion to your art, its importance…and mothers."

Julie craned her neck to stretch, instantly regretting it as pain streaked down her broken arm. After the pain subsided, she said, "I realize it's a double standard, but I can judge for myself whether it's worth the risk to write like Shakespeare."

Pete snorted.

"At least my writing is publishable now. Running a slight risk to my health to write a great novel is worth it."

"And it's not worth it to take a slight risk to play in the NFL in front of 60,000 fans? To win games? To win the Super Bowl? To be rich and famous and remembered?"

"And possibly die. I don't want to lose you, Pete."

"I don't want to lose you, Mom."

They sat in the darkened car, each lost in their own thoughts. A sport utility vehicle drove past behind them taking someone home from another long day of work. Only the widely dispersed parked cars of the nightshift nurses, doctors and support staff were left in the deserted structure.

Pete said, "You can't stop me taking steroids."

"Coach will catch you and kick you off the team for good."

"I know how to get away with it."

"Not last time."

"I was surprised by the test because you made me late."

"So it's my fault?"

Pete shook his head as if she would never understand. He looked at his thick hands in his lap. "I'd do anything to play pro football. It's all I want to do, all I want to be."

"I'd do anything to become a novelist. It's all I want to do, all I want to be." Julie looked over at her son, the movement causing pain to course down her arm through her wrist to her finger tips. She winced and held still. When the pain passed, tired of arguing, she said, "Looks like we're at an impasse, Pete. I don't want you to take steroids."

"I don't want you to take those drugs."

Julie considered, letting her mind wander through the possibilities: none were good. She would have loved to have delayed this, but it could not be delayed. This had to be settled now, when Pete was talking. He might never open up to her again. Taking a deep breath and steeling her nerves, she said, "I'll make a deal with you."

"What?" Pete asked, his eyes narrowing warily.

Julie hesitated, then said before she could stop herself, "You stop taking steroids and I will stop taking the drugs from the trial."

There, she had said it. She already regretted making the offer. She should have just told him not to take steroids, but she knew it wasn't as simple as that. She could not control him like that, not without his cooperation, not any more. The 'Ode on a Grecian Urn' might be worth any number of old ladies, but wasn't worth even one son—not her son.

Pete looked at her, their eyes meeting as each considered what such a deal would mean.

"We could both just keep taking the drugs," Pete suggested. "You could be a novelist and I could play for the Bears. What a life for both of us."

"We could both die before you ever played a single game in college and before my first book ever hit the stores."

Pete leaned back in the car seat and tucked his head down to inspect the fingers of his right hand. "You'll stop taking the drugs right now?"

"Yes, and you stop taking steroids."

After a long, considered pause, Pete nodded, slowly and reluctantly.

*Medicine….does not consist of compounding
pills and plasters; it deals with the very
processes of life, which must be understood
before they may be guided.*

— Paracelsus, Renaissance physician,
1493-1541

Held tight in his right fist, Pete brought his plastic pill bottle of steroids into the kitchen the next morning before breakfast.

"That all of them?" Julie asked as she stood before the white garbage can.

"Yes," Pete said, biting off the word like a curse. "Yours?"

She reached over with her good hand onto the granite counter and picked up a plastic shopping bag. It rattled and jingled as she held it up.

"All of them?"

Julie nodded.

"We don't have to do this."

"We do, Pete. We do."

Julie opened the garbage can.

Pete pursed his lips and turned his head to the side.

"What?" Julie asked.

"Doesn't seem right, just dumping them all."

"Doesn't seem to fit such a dramatic moment in our lives?"

Pete's eyes widened and the hint of a smile touched his lips. He dropped his bottle on the counter and rushed out to the garage. He returned with a hammer and his smile had grown.

"We could just flush them down the toilet," Julie suggested.

"Have you heard about all the drugs they find in the water supply?"

Pete pulled out a wood cutting board and opened his pill bottle. He set a pile of octagonal pills on the board and looked at Julie. She opened her plastic bag and struggled to open a pill container with her good hand. Pete took the container and opened it to add some of her trial drugs to his pile.

Julie sniffed and blinked back the emotions that threatened to engulf her. His body rigid, his face set in a look that would not have been out of place at a funeral of a beloved one, Pete raised the hammer and started to methodically pulverize the steroids and trial drugs.

As much as we watch to see what our children do with their lives, they are watching us to see what we do with ours. I can't tell my children to reach for the sun. All I can do is reach for it myself.

—Joyce Maynard, US author, b. 1953

Pete took his second drug test a week after the first. As he came in the door from school, Julie said, "Coach called. You failed the drug test."

Pete swore.

"The steroids can stay in your system for two or three weeks," Julie told him, but that information did nothing to cheer him up. "Be thankful you weren't injecting the steroids."

"What difference would that make?" Pete asked as he flung himself onto the sofa in the living room.

"Injected steroids can stay in your system for six months or more. Orally, they're expelled within two or three weeks." She paused looking down at him and asked, "You have stopped taking them?"

"Of course," Pete snapped back. "I'm not stupid. I want to get back on the team."

"Are you sure?"

"We have a deal, Mom."

"I'm sticking to our deal, so I hope you are." Julie had hoped that with their deal and the end of the steroids, Pete's mood would stabilize. It had not happened, but should soon, if he had indeed stopped taking them. In either case, he was, she guessed, borderline depressed, not that she was in an objective position to judge. With a broken wrist, a depressed son, absent potential boyfriend, mounting bills, the possible loss of her house, maybe having to move her father, and her dream of becoming a novelist gone, she viewed the world as a bleak, hideous place of pain, torment and destroyed dreams. She struggled just to get out of bed. "I got some information on the negative side effects of steroid use for you."

"I know them all. I won't take steroids, alright? We have a deal. I promised; you promised."

Staring at him a moment, Julie nodded and returned to the kitchen. She slid a store-bought pan of meatloaf into the preheated oven for dinner. The potatoes and string beans were already cooking. With only one good arm she was relegated to cooking the simplest of meals, but at least she was home now to do it. When she had been working, Pete had eaten dinner alone more nights than he ate with her. She struggled to see whatever silver she could discern in the dark cloud of their deal, which had ended her novelist dreams. She rarely saw anything save black and gray.

At least her arm had subsided into a dull ache now, save for an occasional stab of pain to remind her of the break. The pain was not enough for her to take any pain medication, especially since she didn't want Pete to see her taking pills and think she was back on the trial drugs.

Slumped on the sofa, Pete fiddled with one of the straps on his black backpack.

"There's a Bears-Packers game tonight," Julie said, making it sound tempting. The last thing she wanted to do was watch a football game. Her first choice was to crawl into bed and sleep for a month or two, but seeing him so down only worsened her misery.

"I don't have any money on it, Mom," Pete assured her. He sounded dispirited, tired and down.

"I didn't mean," Julie began, then changed course. "I thought maybe we could watch it together like we used to; make popcorn, drink sodas, and yell at the coaches and refs. You'll have to make the popcorn, though." She gestured with her chin at her cast.

Pete nodded glum acceptance of her offer.

"Don't worry, Pete, you'll pass the next drug test."

He nodded, but looked far from convinced.

"You'll get back on the team."

He nodded again, flung a strap on his backpack hard to one side and asked, "How's the novel coming?"

"Slowly."

Julie had dreaded this meeting. She shook with nervousness. Her stomach churned. Arriving at the ocean-view bistro in Carlsbad, her mom and sister offered sympathy for her wrist, although they accepted her story of tripping over a pile of clothes in Pete's room without question. As they finished their meals, Julie decided the time had come. She hadn't touched her teriyaki chicken salad.

She glanced at her mom. Darkly pretty, even in her late sixties, Julie's mom exuded a quiet confidence and a European style. She ate with precision. Her fork speared each piece of precisely sliced miso salmon on her plate and transported it efficiently to her mouth. Then the white linen napkin wiped away any residue of the transaction from her lips. She had never done an impulsive thing in her life, Julie thought. Not ever.

Julie pursed her lips and stared at her sister. Younger, dressed in a low-cut yellow blouse and tight jeans, she had been the flighty sister. She meandered through high school and college with little direction or cares. She was often told she had to find something to do with her life. Then she met perfect Dennis. He worked. She did not. Life solved.

"I left Mount Hermon," Julie said, before she could dwell any more on how best to tell them.

Her mother's silver fork stopped halfway between plate and mouth. Her sister's head cocked to one side with a quizzical expression, as if someone had passed gas at an adjacent table.

"Pardon me?" her mother asked. Her well made-up forehead wrinkled in confusion.

"They let me go." Seeing that they both still stared at her, Julie added, "Fired me, sacked me, told me my services were no longer required, goodbye and good riddance."

"In God's name, why?" her mother asked.

"You're a great doctor," her sister exclaimed, as if it was a universal truth.

Julie had thought the worst was over but now, she realized, came the hard part. For a second, she had an overpowering urge to bolt out of the restaurant, but Pete had driven her down and was visiting friends in Pacific Beach for another hour.

She explained: the drugs, writing like Shakespeare, the agent and the publisher, leaving the OR, missing the call, and being fired.

Her mother and sister stared at her.

"You must be mad," her mother said, her tone even and level, as if she was in a daze.

"Crazy is more like it," her sister said. "Are you insane?"

"No, I want to be a novelist."

"Then write," her mother exclaimed. "Don't risk your life with some silly drugs."

"You gave up your job, all that money, for what?" her sister asked.

"I'm just relieved your father will never know about this," her mother said, placing her fork precisely down beside her plate. "It would break his heart."

"I doubt it," Julie mumbled.

"Pardon me?" her mother asked, taking on that maternal tone all children loathe.

Julie looked up and met her mother's gaze. "I said, I doubt he would be heartbroken. If anything, I think he would understand."

"If you think that, you're further gone than he is," her mother said. "He worked every day of his life since he was 14 years old, 15 and 16 hours a day, building his business. He lived and breathed for that business. He would never do such a silly thing."

"That's exactly why he'd understand."

They stared at her without any comprehension, let alone understanding. Meeting their incredulous stares, Julie realized that they would never understand. It was impossible. It was not her; it was them. Something was lacking in them.

She had planned to broach the other subject she had been stewing about later, but now seemed as good a time as any. "I may need to reduce some costs," she said. "We may need to move Dad to a less expensive nursing home."

Her mother and sister shook their heads, taken aback by the sudden change in the course of the conversation. Neither, Julie knew, thought much about money, especially since Julie often took on major expenses for the extended family from Dad's nursing home to college funds for nieces and nephews, and, two years before, a car for her sister's son for college. Why hadn't perfect Dennis paid for it?

"We can't move him," her mother said, her face set in a stern look Julie recognized as broaching no disagreement. "He's happy there; well taken care of."

"I can't afford it. I—we don't have any choice. I can't stop paying for health insurance for Pete and me, or stop paying my mortgage. Even as it is, if I don't find a job soon, Pete and I will have to move to something cheaper."

"No," her mother gasped. "You love that house. What about Pete?"

"Surely you can manage the mortgage until you find a new job," her sister said, shocked.

"You'll find a position soon," her mother said with a reassuring smile and a pat on Julie's hand.

"Not many neurosurgery positions open and, with Pete, I can't leave Los Angeles. I'll be lucky to find a job in a year and that's if anyone will even give me an interview once they hear the reason Mount Hermon fired me."

"It can't be that bleak," her sister said, frowning as she tried to assimilate this turn of events.

"It is. I made a pile of money, but I was spending a pile of money. When my income stopped, the bills were—are way out of line with what I can afford. My savings are vanishing fast."

"I really don't want to move your father," her mother said, clutching her linen napkin.

"We'll have to," Julie said. "His care is $75,000 a year."

Julie had never seen two such shocked faces.

Julie opened the door the next morning to get the mail from the box at the gate. Instead she found the mail stacked on the doormat. Beside it sat a flat metal kitchen container with a note taped on top; "Heat in 325-degree oven for 15 minutes. I assume you don't eat ham. Homemade. Hope the wrist heals fast. Alan."

Frowning at the container, she bent down and lifted the lid. Inside was a pizza with mozzarella, barbequed chicken and mushrooms covering the top. The sight brought the first smile to her lips since she broke her wrist.

*Remember that you are a human being with
a soul and the divine gift of articulate speech;
that your native language is the language of
Shakespeare and Milton and the Bible; and
don't sit there crooning like a bilious pigeon.*

—George Bernard Shaw

Julie sat in her home office at her laptop, smoking—little compensation for the loss of the trial drugs—and held one of her good fingers poised over the mouse to send the draft of the remainder of her novel to her agent, Charles Wood-Byrd. The first six chapters of the novel had been written under the influence of the drugs, the remainder had not. Rereading it, Julie realized that the difference between the first six chapters and the rest of the novel was as stark as comparing Shakespeare to a Harlequin romance. Julie had spent weeks revising and reworking the later part of the novel, which she had written clean and sober, as it were, but it still paled in comparison to the first six chapters. After rewriting and revising section after section, she had been driven to the conclusion that the two sections would never be on par with each other, unless she did one of two things: rewrote the first part to be as weak as the second part, which meant it would never be published, or took the trial drugs again. She knew she could not do the later; she and Pete had a deal. The thought struck her like a slap: her ability to write like Shakespeare was gone, and gone forever.

With a resigned sigh, she clicked the send button.

Sitting in the doctor's office waiting for the cardiologist to finish with Pete, Julie felt that depictions of hell had it all wrong. There was no need for fire, lava, devils, racks or any other torture devices. All that was required for hell was to have your child seriously ill or even be suspected of having a serious illness. The thought of something wrong with Pete made her nauseous, dizzy and faint. She could not imagine life without him. There would be no life without him.

Against Pete's protests, Julie had arranged to have their livers, kidneys, lungs, brains, GI tracts, and every other major organ and bodily system, as well as their bones checked. The heart check had been the last thing on her exhaustive list. She had arranged to have them see Dr. Oginweyle, a nationally known cardiologist. Removing an acoustic neuroma from Oginweyle's niece the year before still provided a great deal of pull with the esteemed cardiologist. Julie and Pete had been put through stress tests, cardiac CTs, EKGs, Holter monitor testing and ultrasounds to analyze the condition of their hearts. Today they would learn the results of all the tests.

Julie looked around the office, the tan fabric-covered chairs, the square tables with ordered magazines, and the posters explaining the rights of patients and billing procedures in four languages. The type was so tiny, you would have had sore feet by the time you read it all. The mundane details of hell.

She glanced at her watch. Had the little hand moved at all since she last checked the time?

Tom had wanted to come but she'd said there would be no point. She promised to call him as soon as she knew anything. Now, glancing at an older couple on the other side of the waiting room whispering to each other in their private world, she wished she had let him come. Hell alone had to be worse than hell with someone, even an ex-husband. At least her arm in its enormous cast rarely hurt now save for a most annoying itch every once in a while.

The inner door opened and a nurse beckoned Julie inside, before leading her to a clinic room. Inside Pete sat perched on an exam table in his blue jeans and a T-shirt, while Oginweyle, a large, black Barbados native, sat on a low, black, wheeled stool. Julie sat on a gray plastic chair.

"Pete has some slight damage I'd like to keep an eye on with another checkup in six months," Oginweyle said.

"What about football?" Pete asked.

"I don't see any indications why you shouldn't be able to play," Oginweyle said. "The arrhythmia appears to have been caused by the steroid use. There is slight damage to one of the valves, but it shouldn't be a problem for years, if ever."

Julie nodded, relieved beyond measure.

"And you," Oginweyle said, swiveling toward Julie. "Your heart appears fine. A little plaque, but normal for your age, if not a little better than average. I'd keep up the cardio workouts, jogging, though."

The tension drained from Julie's body and a wave of exhaustion washed over her.

With the results from his third drug test, which showed no drugs, a letter from his mother, another from his father, and Pete's heartfelt promise never to take steroids again, Coach Paukenan allowed Pete to rejoin the team's practice squad. Pete would not play—not even as a substitute tight end—until it was clear that he was not going to take steroids again. Pete asked how long that would be, but all Coach Paukenan would say was, "I'll let you know."

In the meantime, the weekly drug tests continued and Pete suffered the ignominy of wearing the white practice T-shirt of a non-starter, instead of the dark-green practice jersey of a starter, which he had worn for three straight years. He felt humiliated putting on the stark, white shirt, but he sucked it up, channeling his anger into training and practicing harder than anyone else so he could regain a coveted dark-green jersey as fast as possible.

"You'll be back soon," Manny Ortiz told him as they walked out to practice one afternoon. Manny wore the white shirt of a backup, but his back was straight and his chest was out.

Pete grunted an acknowledgement.

After practice, the players gathered around Coach Paukenan. "Starting linebackers for Friday are Jayden Andrews and Joe Cain," Paukenan announced. Pete knew it was coming, but it still hurt.

Coach didn't even look at him. Once you were off the first string, you were forgotten, like an old pair of shoes.

As the rest of the players streamed back across the playing fields toward the locker room, Pete started a series of blocking drills alone. If he couldn't take steroids, he would have to work twice as hard as anyone else. If practice was an hour and a half, he would stay to work out another hour and a half by himself. He would regain his spot on the team; he had to.

He lined up on a blocking sled and, slamming into the padded arm, drove the sled back with tired legs thirty feet. He rested a few moments and did it again, and again, driving the sled the length of the field. Then he slid the sled around and drove it back the length of the field in the other direction.

Taking a long drink of water from a plastic bottle, Pete scanned the darkening sky and decided he should work on his stamina. Shoulder pads clicking and clacking, he started jogging around the track. A brief storm blew in off the Pacific, drenching him in a fast-moving rain burst, but it merely darkened his uniform more evenly than it had been with his own sweat.

If you train hard, you'll not only be hard,
you'll be hard to beat.

—Herschel Walker, US football player, b. 1962

December

Pete crouched, heard an imaginary count in his head and on the second 'hike!' launched himself down the track in a determined 40-yard dash. Just as Adina had taught him, he kept his legs vertical and his arms pumping evenly as he accelerated down the cinder track. He slowed after 40 yards and turned to trot back and try it again.

"Good form!"

Surprised, Pete looked over and spotted Adina. He nodded his thanks for the compliment. He hadn't seen her since he'd been kicked off the team. He was sure everyone in the school knew why: steroids, and being dumb enough to get caught. The latter was far worse in the eyes of most of the other students than the former.

"Heard you're back on the team," Adina said, striding over toward him, her long, jeans-clad legs covering the distance with an easy, flowing grace as if she was made of a fine, dark liquid.

"I'm not allowed to play in any games yet."

"If you keep working as hard as you've been, you should be soon. I've seen you out here every day." She stopped before him and added with a smile, "You look good."

Pete didn't know if she was referring to his sprinting form or his looks, but he knew that his acne had cleared up and his hair was fuller again.

"I'm just trying to keep training every day and focus on getting back into a game."

"You sound down," Adina said as they meandered back toward the starting line for his next sprint.

Pete managed a grin. "The doctor said after you stop taking…. well, you tend to get mood swings."

"The steroids produce testosterone and your body stops producing it," Adina said. "When you stop taking them, your body doesn't realize it has to restart producing testosterone for a while, so mood swings are common."

Surprised, Pete stopped and stared at Adina.

"Steroids are pretty common in track," she said. "My parents wanted to make sure I didn't take any, so they had me read all about them."

"Did it work?"

"It did."

Pete wondered why he had taken steroids even when he knew the risks. Maybe he just wanted to be a pro football player more than Adina wanted to run track.

"How did you do so well without help?" he asked.

"Hard work, just like you're doing now."

"But you compete against girls who must take steroids."

"They compete against someone who practices twice as much as they do." She hesitated, glanced over at the deserted school and asked, "If you've done enough for today, would you like to go get a coffee or tea or something?"

Pete knew he should practice for another half hour, but her bright smile changed his mind. "Sure."

Now that she had made the deal with Pete, Julie regretted not stopping taking the drugs earlier, submitting to the drug tests to keep her position at Mount Hermon, and maybe not losing Alan. Had she lost him? Even though prepared food had appeared on her porch a dozen times, she hadn't seen Alan in weeks. She considered going over to visit, but feared what he would say.

She considered calling Dr. Baxter and asking whether she might be considered for her old position—with drug tests, of course, but she could not bring herself to make the call. Her pride, self esteem and the conclusion that he would in all likelihood refuse, dissuaded her from calling him for a letter of recommendation, let alone a job. She also realized that what she really regretted was that she had been unable to stay on the drugs long enough to finish her novel.

As she struggled to look for a job online with her good hand, she found positions for internists, GPs and entry-level physicians in various clinics and hospitals around Los Angeles, but no openings for a neurosurgeon. Even so, she had to find a job so she applied to every position for which she was even remotely qualified.

She tried to brighten her outlook by daydreaming that Wood-Byrd would love her novel, Jonathan Sharpe would publish it and it would become a bestseller. She had visions of a national book tour, radio and television interviews, a spot on Oprah, and the adoration of millions of readers. Most of all, she dreamed of a writing life: able to support herself and Pete by writing, by making up stories and writing them down. What a wonderful life it would be.

If it ever was to be, she had better start her next novel. Beginning on a new blank screen on her laptop, she started pecking out a three-page outline with one hand, re-read it, groaned, erased it and tried again. Again, crap. Staring at the blank screen, she wondered what drove her to do this. Why had she been cursed with the desire to take 26 letters and in endless variations turn them into stories for other people to read? She knew she had something to say. She had stories to tell. She just had to tell them well; to tell them perfectly. Why was it so hard?

"Linebackers for Friday's last game of the regular season," Coach Paukenan announced, pausing in his delivery as Pete turned away at the end of yet another grueling practice. Pete was headed to the track to run laps to start his private, post-practice training regimen. This announcement would not concern him.

"Jayden Andrews and, for busting his ass, Pete Tomlinson."

Mediocrity knows nothing higher than itself;
but talent instantly recognizes genius...

—Sir Arthur Conan Doyle

One cool December day as Julie struggled with her new novel, the doorbell chimed. It was Alan, clutching her novel chapters.

Alan said, "I read your book." He held up her sample chapters. "At least the part you gave me."

She nodded, glad he had come, but wondering with trepidation whether he would understand. Would he think she was insane? Would he like her novel?

"You said you were fired for taking drugs to write it?" Alan asked. He spoke slowly. His face was set in a serious expression and his eyes focused on Julie.

She nodded and explained the relationship she suspected between the drugs in her clinical trial and creativity.

"I like the chapters, but it still seems a bizarre thing to do," Alan said, choosing his words with care. "To be honest, at first I was worried and considered calling someone to commit you."

"I want to be a novelist and I wasn't publishing anything without the drugs."

"You want to be a writer that much?"

"More than anything."

"You risked your health."

"I know."

"And your job."

"I love writing. Nothing else even comes close; nothing. I have to write. If I don't, I feel as if...as if I'm not alive."

He nodded, sucked on his lower lip and said, "After I read the chapters, I wondered if they were really good."

"I thought you liked them."

"I don't mean just good to me—a casual reader—but good to a real writer, someone who knows what good writing is. So I showed your chapters to a friend of mine. He's the one I mentioned, who retired and writes military-techno thrillers. I hope you don't mind."

She shook her head. The porch was quiet. She heard the wind rustling a palm across the street. She smelled smoke from a fireplace on the breeze.

"He said it was some of the best writing he's ever read."

"An agent in New York and a publisher are interested in it, too," Julie said, the words tumbling out in a rush. "They want to publish it." At least she hoped they still did.

"That's fantastic."

They stood beaming at each other. He looked down at the chapters in his hand. After a long moment, he said, "I think I understand why you did it."

"I'm relieved."

"I still don't think you should have done it, but I understand—I think." He looked over at her, his face wearing an expression of concern and confusion. "I'm just relieved you stopped taking the drugs."

Julie nodded, a cauldron of conflicting emotions roiling within her. She had lost her job, her potential boyfriend and almost her son to the drugs that had let her write like Shakespeare, yet, even now, she doubted whether she would have done anything differently, except hide her drug taking more effectively.

"I can only imagine what damage the drugs were doing to your body," Alan said. "Nothing's worth that."

Julie wondered if saving a fellow soldier's life was worth that to him, but didn't ask—the medals on his wall provided a clear answer.

I've missed more than 9,000 shots in my career. I've lost almost 300 games. Twenty-six times I've been trusted to take the game winning shot and missed. I've failed over and over and over again in my life and that is why I succeed.

—Michael Jordan, US basketball player, b. 1963

Filled with adrenaline and focused on playing well in his first game back since his drug suspension, Pete slid to the right just as the center hiked the ball. Pete guessed that the Windsor Lions would try a screen pass to the short side.

The Lions' quarterback rolled back to Pete's left, drawing the defense after him. Pete held back, drifting farther over to his right. A wide receiver slid in from near the sideline to block for a running back who was swinging out to the short side right in front of Pete.

As the quarterback swiveled his head to throw to the running back over the onrushing defensive players, Pete put his sprint training to good use. He cut between the would-be blocking receiver and the running back. As the back caught the ball, Pete wrapped his arms around his legs three yards behind the line of scrimmage. A perfect play.

Even though Pete hit him going fast and hard, the back stayed on his feet. Pete dug in his cleats to finish the tackle, but the power back was not going down. He spun and twisted. Before Pete knew it, the back wrenched free of his embrace. Pete was left lying on the turf as the back raced up field behind his receiver-blocker.

The sophomore safety, Manny Ortiz raced over. He faked left to avoid the wide-receiver blocker and shoved the back out of bounds, saving a touchdown.

"Pussies should stay at home with their momma's," the running back taunted Pete as the Lion jogged back toward his huddle.

"Fuck you," Pete spat back.

Julie and Alan sat in the stands, three rows below Tom and Christy. Fresh from surgery, Julie's arm was in a smaller post-operative cast. Even so, her wrist could still on occasion make her wince with sudden, sharp pains.

"Tough play," Alan commented.

"He should have had him," Julie said.

"Hard when it's just you." Alan offered Julie some of the hot buttered popcorn he had purchased from a stand run by students.

"That's what middle linebackers are paid to do."

"This is high school, isn't it?" Alan asked, raising an eyebrow at her seriousness.

Julie grinned. "Yeah, but it's just as serious as college or the pros."

"Who knew you were such a football mother."

"If you had a son playing football, you'd be too…well at least a football father."

"He's made a couple of fine tackles."

"On wide receivers, but he's having trouble with the bigger running backs." Julie wondered whether the steroids could have made such a difference. She knew the answer; they had. Otherwise, no one would take them.

In as a tight end, Pete ran a square-out pattern. Running full speed toward the sidelines, he glanced back over his shoulder. The Spartans quarterback, Aaron Stevens looked left. Stevens looked back at Pete and threw the football over an onrushing lineman right at Pete.

Seeing a safety angling across the field toward him out of the corner of his eye, Pete focused on the ball. He reached out and plucked it out of the air. He turned up field just as the safety slammed into his legs. Pete spun up into the air, rolled and slammed into the grass. It was only as he landed that he realized his hands were empty. The safety had stripped the ball. A Lion dove on the ball. How the hell had that happened?

"Hang onto the fucking ball, Tomlinson," Stevens yelled as the Spartans offensive players trudged toward the sidelines. "Since when can a safety take the ball outta your hands?"

In on defense a few minutes later, Pete read the play as a hand-off, with the running back coming up the middle. The quarterback handed the power back the ball. Pete roamed behind his own line, waiting for the back to commit to a slot in the line to burst through.

The back sliced between the center and the right tackle. He cradled the ball with both hands to eliminate any chance of a fumble. Pete slammed into him just as he emerged from the maelstrom of bodies where the two lines were locked in battle. The back was coming at him low, but Pete stood the back up.

A test of strength, Pete and the power back drove their legs into the turf to get traction to drive the other back. After a second of equilibrium, Pete felt himself pushed back and then toppled over. Breaking the tackle, the back burst into the Spartans' backfield.

Furious with himself, Pete scrambled up in hot pursuit. Jayden cut across the field at full speed. Even as Pete sprinted to catch the loose back, Jayden tackled the back from the side, bringing him down with ease.

"Tomlinson! Tomlinson!"

Pete heard Coach Paukenan's angry yells. Pete trotted, head down, over to the sideline.

"Cain in!"

Pete slowed at the sideline, hating to leave the field, and slunk past the coach.

"When you wrap 'em up, you gotta take 'em down," Paukenan ordered, slapping Pete on the back of the helmet as he went by. "You're tackling like a five-year-old girl!"

Pete wrenched off his helmet and threw himself down at the end of the bench, far from the other players. His elbows on his knees, he dropped his helmet and cradled his head in his hands. He cursed the day the drug test had revealed his secret. He cursed his mother for delaying him that fateful morning. He cursed the deal with his mother. If he was on steroids, he would still be playing great. He should take them again. Would she ever know? He had to take them again. He'd never stay on the team, let alone make college or the NFL without them.

He swore.

He could not. He must not. When his mom noticed—how could he hide the effects of the drugs?—she'd take her drugs again. He could not risk losing his mother, let alone be responsible for her death.

As he sat alone, sweat dripped from his face, which was just as well, since it made it so no one could tell he was crying.

The next day, Julie received the letter. The agent did not even do her the kindness of a phone call. Once you were no longer worth anything to them, you were nothing, graciousness be damned. The letter from Charles Wood-Byrd said that regrettably the novel, which had shown such great promise, failed to carry through to the conclusion with the same high level of readability. Wood-Byrd was terribly sorry, but Jonathan Sharpe and Kira House Press had declined to accept it for publication and, Charles wrote, he did not feel confident trying to place it at any other publishing house. He wished her well finding another agent who would better be able to represent her and her novel.

Julie wandered out onto the back deck in a daze. In the waning light of a cool, late autumn day, she lit a cigarette. She wished she could take the drugs from her trial again. It would be so easy; to write so well, to publish novels, to fulfill her dream and to be great.

She could not. Pete would find it. How could she hide the effects? He would start taking steroids again. She could not risk Pete's life. As she faced the cost of the deal she had made with Pete, she cried.

*The ultimate decision about what is accepted
as right and wrong will be made not by
individual human wisdom but by the
disappearance of the groups that have
adhered to the 'wrong' beliefs.*

—Fredrich August von Hayek, economist,
Nobel Laureate, 1899-1992

Hanukkah passed without notice. Julie lacked the energy to celebrate and, she told herself, Pete was too old for the holiday anyways. She missed the years when he had been young and loved playing dreidel, lighting the menorah, eating latkes and devouring candy. Those days seemed so long ago. She had been busy then, but had had far more energy. Now she was tired all the time and Pete, after his poor performance in the last football game, was in no mood to celebrate anything.

Pete sat in his bedroom holding his cell phone. He clicked through his address book until he came to the science geek Mike's number. Pete stared down at the name glowing on the tiny screen, considering, weighing and wondering. He saw himself in a Bears uniform, sprinting onto Soldier Field to the roar of the sell-out crowd. In his mind, he looked over toward the stands and spotted his cheering father. Then he saw his mother. She looked on with grim disapproval as she shook her head.

"Shit," he said and clicked the phone off. He had given his word.

"Eight seconds left. Vikings on the Spartans' 3-yard line." Excitement drove the announcer's voice at the Carson Center. "The Spartans' defense was caught napping on this drive. It's 14-10 Spartans, but they better wake up or they could hand the LA City Championship to the Vikings from Culver City.

"Vikings up to the line; three receivers on the left, one on the right, empty backfield. Spartans showing blitz; their fast linebackers, Joe Cain and Jayden Andrews rush up to the line. Arnold snaps the ball.

"Cain comes on the blitz. Jayden holds back.

"Sanderson drops back. Cain squeezes through a hole in the Viking line. Sanderson looks for a receiver; they're blanketed. He pumps, but holds onto the ball.

"Cain forces Sanderson out of the pocket. He grabs Sanderson's jersey. Sanderson twists, breaks free and sets to throw.

"The Vike's Rashad comes across the back of the end zone, covered by the Spartans' Eihorn. Rashad has a step on Eihorn. Sanderson throws just as Cain brings him down. Rashad has it!

"No, no, he doesn't. Jayden came flying in and delivered a punishing hit on Rashad. Rashad dropped the ball. The officials rule he never had possession.

"Time has run out. The Santa Maria Spartans have stopped the Culver City Vikings and won the Los Angeles City High School Football Championship!"

Pete sat on a metal bench on the sidelines alone. At the start of the game, against all hope, he had paced the sidelines, ready, eager and desperate to play. He stayed close to Coach Paukenan, praying Paukenan would send him in. At halftime, Pete had tried to catch Paukenan's eye without success. By the end of the third quarter Pete sat despondent on the bench, all hope gone. And now before him, all his teammates flooded onto the field. Yelling, screaming and tackling each other with joy, the Spartans celebrated their victory. Players doused coaches with barrels of orange, sticky sport drink while other players hoisted Cain and Jayden, the heroes of the game, onto their shoulders to carry the pair to the center of the field for the trophy presentation.

Pete thumped his clean helmet hard onto the turf between his feet. His immaculate uniform and the gleaming white tape on his hands and around his ankles remained unsullied by contact with the field. They shone as badges of failure for all to see.

"Did you get your shirt and ring?"

Dazed, Pete looked up at Manny Ortiz, the sophomore safety. Ortiz wore a white Spartans football T-shirt that proclaimed them LA City Champions. Manny held out a shirt and a heavy, bronze ring to Pete.

"It's just a temporary ring," Manny explained. He couldn't stand still from the excitement. "We'll get our real ones later."

"I don't get one," Pete said, his voice bitter.

"Course you do. You're on the team, just like me."

"Did you play tonight?" Pete snapped.

The excitement vanished from Manny's body as he lowered the offered shirt and ring.

Seeing the effect of his words, Pete added, "I didn't play either."

Manny nodded. "I'll just leave them here."

Setting the shirt and precious ring carefully on the bench beside Pete, Manny started toward the center of the field where the Spartans players, coaches, cheerleaders and a horde of students celebrated with wild abandon.

Pete glared down at the shirt with the ring perched atop it.

Manny stopped and called back, "You deserve it."

"No, I don't."

"You played most of the season. You averaged 13 tackles a game. You're an important part of the team."

Pete grabbed the shirt and ring and, flinging them into the large, plastic garbage can at the end of the bench, yelled, "Not anymore" and stalked off toward the locker room alone.

The best way to appreciate your job
is to imagine yourself without one.

—Oscar Wilde

February

Too early one morning, Julie's cell buzzed on her bedside table.

"This is Deborah Wright at the South LA Free Clinic," a rapid, efficient voice said. "I'm sorry to call at the crack of dawn, but I thought I'd take a chance. One of our physicians just passed away."

"I'm sorry to hear that," Julie said as she tried to figure out why this woman, who she vaguely remembered from volunteering at the clinic, was calling her to tell her some doctor she had never heard of had died.

"Fell off a mountain in Alaska."

"How terrible," Julie said.

"He's left us with a full slate of patients and no doctor to see them," Wright continued as if Julie hadn't said a word. "All our other physicians are already seeing more patients than they should."

"Oh," Julie managed to say for lack of anything better as she blinked sleep out of her eyes.

"I heard via the physician grapevine that you were looking for a position and, I know it's far from neurosurgery and we can't pay much—$200 a day to start—but we desperately need a GP."

Julie was now fully awake. Her savings were gone. The next mortgage payment loomed and her father's nursing home bill would arrive in the mail any day. "For how long?"

"As long as you want to stay."

"My wrist isn't one hundred percent," Julie said, deciding honesty was the best way to start a new position. "I broke it in the fall." With intensive physio she was approaching the full range of motion and old level of strength in her wrist and fingers, but they still throbbed and went numb at least once a day, and her thumb was almost always stiff. Her physio was confident that with time and diligent exercise of the fingers, wrist and thumb Julie soon would be able to perform neurosurgical procedures.

"Can you use your hand enough to see patients in clinic? We don't need a surgeon, just a general practitioner."

"I think so."

"I'm willing to give it a go, if you are."

Julie bit her lip. Working as a GP in a clinic was far from what she wanted to do, but it was a job and it sounded like she was needed.

"When do you need someone?"

"Can you be here for 8 a.m. clinic?"

Julie dragged herself through her front door at 9 p.m. Fighting to keep her eyes open, she checked her cell phone messages and heard one from Pete; he was going out for dinner with a friend. No name, as usual. At least he didn't sound as down as he had in recent days.

Julie crawled over to the fridge, saw nothing that appealed and just made it to her bed before collapsing. She had seen 52 patients in 12 hours at the clinic, everything from an ear infection and fractured finger to diabetes and a possible bone tumor. After a few months off work and with her body worn down by the drugs she had taken, she felt as if she'd just swum the Pacific while towing the *Queen Mary* behind her. Her wrist was throbbing and she hoped she had not damaged it again. It was probably just fatigue.

She managed to stand to undress. Through tired, blurry eyes, she peered at her jogging shoes in the closet. The sneakers had not been used in quiet some time. They would not be used tonight or probably the next morning either. She had to be at the clinic at first light and if her body felt even only half as bad as it did now, she couldn't manage to jog across her bedroom, let alone a few miles. The LA Marathon would not be on her agenda this year.

She considered writing, but her body rebelled at the thought. She knew she had to write for her mental health. If she did not write, she would become clinically depressed. She took a step toward her home office, stopped and, teetering, fell back onto the bed. Maybe tomorrow.

By late February, Julie finished a short story she had written in stolen moments during lunch at the clinic and late at night at home. She had thought about revising the novel she had started under the influence of the trial drugs, but after several attempts to improve the second part to match the first in terms of quality, she had given up. The quality was so different it was as if it had been written by two different people. She was tempted to take the trial drugs to finish the novel, but she feared Pete finding out. She could not risk him taking steroids again. With football season over, there would be no random drug test to catch him if he did. She had to rely on their deal and, if she didn't keep her part of it, how could she expect him to? She submitted the short story to 10 literary journals.

Julie decided she had to start getting back into shape. The clinic job was killing her and, with such long days, it left little time for anything else. Now that she was learning how to see patients more efficiently, as well as mastering the reams of paperwork involved, she was getting home closer to 6 than to 8. This meant that she had an hour or two after dinner when she could write. The problem was that her body wasn't up to it. If she got into better shape, she hoped she would be able to write more, and write more effectively.

The next morning with the sun just cresting the horizon, she was jogging along her street after returning from an abbreviated run when a voice called out, "Been a while."

She turned and saw Alan McGhee picking up his *Los Angeles Times* on his front steps. He walked with no sign of a limp. Macduff rutted around in the yard, barking at a passing pick-up.

Julie changed course and forced her aching legs to carry her up to Alan. Macduff paraded over to say hello, wagging his tail and accepting scratches behind his regal ears. Julie appeared to still be on his short list of friends.

"Your leg's healed?" Julie asked between puffs as she caught her breath. She was in awful shape. Her legs were flabby and she dared not even consider the state of her butt.

Alan lifted his leg off the ground and bent it back and forth as if it was a new toy. "Good as new. A little stiff in the morning, but if I keep doing the 15 hours worth of exercises the physio gave me to do every day, it should be 100 percent within the week," he said with a grin. "How's your wrist?"

"Healed."

"A little faster than a knee."

"Falling against a wall is a lot less traumatic than being hit by a rocket-propelled grenade."

"True, but the RPG makes a better story. Coffee?"

"I can't, sorry. I'm working at a clinic now and," glancing at her watch, "I have to get going as soon as I get cleaned up."

"Dinner?"

Julie froze at the unexpected invitation. What did he mean? Dinner out? At his house? Even as her mind raced through the question's possible meanings, she realized that she didn't care what he meant. "Sure, but it's on me. I still owe you for all the meals that magically appeared on my doorstep when my wrist was broken."

"If that's the case, what's the most expensive restaurant in town?"

By the following spring, with the previous director having moved to direct a medical group in Austin, Texas, Julie had been promoted to medical director of the free clinic. She still longed to find a neurosurgery position but none had come open in the area. If she was to return to neurosurgery she would have to do it soon before her neurosurgical board certification expired. With no recent surgeries or publications, she would be hard pressed to be re-certified if she lost her certification and she dreaded the thought of having to re-sit the rigorous board exams. With Pete's graduation only two months away, she decided to start applying to neurosurgical positions across the country. She had accepted that soon he would be on his own and so would she. There was still the problem of explaining to a new employer her sudden departure from Mount Hermon, but she hoped that someone would at least give her a chance to explain.

After months on a reduced income, she had also faced the fact that something major had to change. With a choice between their home and her father, she had been forced with a great reluctance to choose her son over her father. This would be her father's last month in his current nursing home. She had done extensive research online, made dozens of phone calls and checked several nursing home association rating lists. She had found an excellent full-care facility in Escondido, just inland from Carlsbad, which cost half what the home in Carlsbad charged. She dreaded the move, but she had to do it. Her sister and mother had been willing to chip in some money, but far from enough to make up for Julie's sudden decrease in income. Julie announced her decision at a family dinner and her mother and sister didn't talk to her for a month.

Julie was still writing, submitting stories and novel chapters to magazines, agents and publishers. The rejection file, which she had once kept at work, now resided in a file cabinet in her home office. It had thickened with monotonous regularity. Purim provided a relief of sorts when she invited Alan to come with her and Pete to her sister's house. By then she was no longer persona non grata in the family. Alan got into the spirit of making noise with Julie's young nieces and nephews at every mention of Haman's name, the villain who planned to exterminate the Jews, but was foiled by Esther so long ago. For all the fun, the next morning Julie still hadn't published anything and she still faced another grueling week at the clinic.

Success is the ability to go from one failure to another with no loss of enthusiasm.

—Winston Churchill

June

Pete sat slumped in his black gown at graduation, exhausted, frustrated and on the edge of depression, yet with an undercurrent of nervous excitement. He had already been to parties on three consecutive nights. The ceremony was this afternoon and the formal was that evening. He spotted Adina, just ending her junior year, in the crowd of parents, family and friends in the steamy, packed auditorium. The air conditioning was unable to handle the capacity crowd of excited students and spectators on a hot southern California night.

"Turning to football scholarships," announced Principal Ed Maverly, who reminded Pete of a stork. Pete tuned in to the principal at the mention of his sport. "We have several students who have done well, just as our team did this year, winning the Los Angeles City Championship."

The crowd roared and applauded. Pete lowered his head and tried not to think back to that horrible night.

"Several players are on their way to top collegiate programs across the country," Maverly continued, pride clear in his voice.

Pete heard several teammates' names and then, "Jayden Andrews is following in his father's footsteps to play on a full scholarship for the University of Nebraska." Applause. "Our other All-State linebacker, Joe Cain, has signed to attend the University of Texas, near his hometown, also on a full scholarship."

Pete had heard rumors that Jayden and Cain both had off-campus apartments, cars and jobs already lined up. They made it sound as if all they had to do was play football and show up at the jobs once every couple of weeks to pick up a paycheck. Even if it was only half as sweet as they boasted, they sounded well set on their way to the NFL. Pete sighed; all of it could have been his for the taking.

Pete tuned out as several more of his former teammates were lauded for their scholarships to top college football programs from Washington to Florida and Virginia Tech to Notre Dame. With a wave of anger and profound sadness, he recalled the sudden decrease in the number of phone calls and letters from college coaches after his failed drug test and then the complete absence of any communications after he finally made it back into a game, only to play so poorly. The drug test could have been handled; not playing well could not. When Pete called two of the coaches who had shown great interest in him earlier in the year, one was out all the time and the other, when Pete reached him after weeks of trying, said that he didn't think Pete was up to the standards required for college football.

Cain had 13.8 tackles per game, Jayden 13.6 and Pete 12.9 in his shortened season, his numbers hurt by his performance in his last game. Less than one tackle per game was the difference between a full free ride to the University of Nebraska and nothing.

"Peter Moshe Tomlinson," the principal announced.

Julie watched her drawn and pale son in his somber black gown trudge across the stage to accept his diploma. Pete shook hands with the principal. Whereas all the other graduates had shown great emotion and excitement, many turning to the crowd with arms raised or at least a broad smile of glee, Pete glanced at the audience with a glum expression and slunk off the stage as if headed to his own execution.

"He seems pretty beat," Alan commented. In gray slacks and a dark blue shirt, he looked the picture of an aristocratic gentleman with his straight back and short-cropped hair. "Too many parties?

"Depressed," Julie said.

"Why?"

"He wanted a football scholarship more than anything else in the world." She paused and was about to say, 'And I took it away from him,' but could not say it. She knew it was not her fault. She had done the right thing. She knew she had.

The next morning, Julie arose to have breakfast and found a note on the kitchen table. Pete must have scribbled it when he had come home to change after the formal before he headed out to the various after-parties with Adina. He hadn't wanted to go to any of them but after Julie had failed to convince him, Adina had managed to get him to go.

"Mom," Julie read, "I'm sorry I didn't win any scholarships. I tried my best and I don't have anyone to blame but myself. I will work hard to try and make you proud. Pete."

Julie sat down, sighed and reread the note. She prayed that he knew she was already more proud of him than anything else in her life.

Academe, n.; An ancient school where morality
and philosophy were taught.
Academy, n.; A modern school were football is
taught.

—Ambrose Bierce, US writer, journalist and
editor, 1842-1914

September

Pete sat in freshman English and wondered what he was doing
there. Staring out the window on the top floor of Weingart Hall, he
could just see the sunlit playing fields at the bottom of the sloped
Occidental College campus. On a whim he had applied to Occidental in Eagle Rock, just west of Pasadena, on the last day for
applications. They accepted him and with little thought he decided
to attend. Whitman College, the University of Nevada, Reno and
Oregon had all accepted him, but without football, he had no interest in any of them. At least Oxy was close to home.

The football team was running blocking drills on the fields.
Even from afar, Pete could see that they were no division 1A team.
They were smaller, slower and far less talented than the teams that
played on television every Saturday in the fall. Even so, a part of
him longed to be out there with them.

The professor, who reminded Pete of a sleepy black bear, asked,
"What do you think the author is saying in this section?"

An eager Latina raised her hand. Pete noticed she was wearing a skin-tight dress that showed off her tanned legs. The prof gestured at her with a paw of a hand.

"I think the author meant that happiness is easy to get, but that being content is much more difficult."

"Can you explain that a little more," the prof prompted.

"I mean, like, you can eat ice cream every day, watch your favorite TV show or text your friends all the time and be happy, but it's fleeting. If you want to be content with your life, then, like, you have to achieve something that's important to you, you know?"

A week later, Pete stood on the football field at Occidental in pads and black helmet. In response to his mom's nagging, he had approached the coach, who agreed to a late tryout for Pete against Oxy's second string. Pete hated the idea. He didn't want to play football anymore, especially not for a school that played in the SCIAC; not exactly the PAC-10. If he could not be one of the best, why bother?

Yet now, standing on the field in full Oxy Tigers regalia, he felt energized, back in his native element. He belonged on a football field.

"Hike!"

The pudgy center snapped the ball and the quarterback handed off to a skinny running back. Pete bounced along the line as the back sought an opening. The back found it and turned up field. Pete rushed into the same gap. Pete collided with the back and wrapped him up, stopping him cold—for a glorious instant.

The wiry back spun, dug in his cleats and broke the tackle, leaving Pete sprawled on his back on the grass.

In the locker room, Pete stripped off his pads, throwing them into the locker that had been assigned to him, at least for a few hours. He didn't need to wait for the coach's verdict. He knew what it would be. He couldn't even stop a second-string back at a third-rate football school like Occidental.

Pete changed into his jeans and a T-shirt, then jammed his wallet and keys into his pockets. Holding his cell phone, he flipped it open. Mike's number at the Ivy League college he was attending back east was on it. Mike had sent it along just in case Pete needed some pharmaceutical help on the field. Pete stared down at the phone. He needed help. He could at least play at Oxy. He could tackle, catch passes as a tight end, and play on Saturdays. It would be fun. It wasn't USC, but it was football.

The deal with his mom popped into his head. Since his father left, he had looked after her. He had checked that the doors were locked every night when they went to bed. He had gone shopping with her if she went after dinner when it was dark. He had protected her. He could not stop now.

With a grimace, he cursed, snapped shut the cell and stalked out of the locker room.

*Your school may have done away with winners
and losers, but life has not.*

—Bill Gates, US entrepreneur, b. 1955

January

Pete's grades arrived in a gray envelope from Occidental College.

"How'd you do?" Julie asked as Pete ripped open the envelope at dinner.

Pete grimaced. With a sullen look, he handed the single sheet to Julie: Bs and Cs.

"You could study a little more."

"Yeah," he said, digging into his mashed potatoes. He appeared disinterested.

"It's important, Pete."

"I know."

"You don't sound like you do," Julie said, fed up with his attitude after a fall full of lackadaisical attention to his classes. "College is goddamn important. It'll determine your future job and whether you succeed at anything else in your life."

Pete threw his fork down on the table with a clatter. "It's boring."

"All of it?"

"Yeah."

"Doesn't any subject interest you?"

Pete grabbed his spoon and pushed a sweat-and-sour meatball around his plate.

"Biology?" Julie prompted.

"No."

"Chemistry?"

"You like those."

"English?"

"No."

"History? You used to love reading books about the Vietnam War."

"Nah."

Julie sighed. She never expected to have this problem with her child. She loved learning. Pete had devoured books as a little boy, but his interest in books waned in his teenaged years and now he would rather eat a book than read one.

"Why don't you try out for their football team next year?" Julie suggested, hoping she could get him interested in something, anything again.

"I didn't make it this year, why would I stand a chance next year?"

"You would if you started training now."

"I'd never make the pros, unless…."

"You are not going to take steroids again. We made a deal."

"I know, I know. You don't have to remind me. I think about it every time I see the team practicing."

Julie looked at him, gauging his pain and loss. He hadn't even watched football on TV in months. Their deal had cost him his world. "Making our deal was the most adult thing you've ever done."

Pete snorted.

"No, I mean it," Julie insisted. "When you're an adult, you'll learn there are more important things in life than yourself and your dreams and goals, especially your family. Sometimes you have to sacrifice for them and I know that you did; you sacrificed for me."

He still looked sullen and angry.

Julie said, "Sometimes I think you gave up more than I did."

"Why?" he spat.

"Young dreams are harder to abandon than old ones."

"Why?"

"Young dreams are filled with a lot more hope."

Pete remained silent, glaring down at his meatballs, now poking at one with his fork as if it was a week-old egg. Julie didn't know what else to say.

After a few minutes, Pete began, "Maybe..."

"What?" Julie lunged at the faint ray of hope from her son.

"PE."

"Physical education?" Julie asked, frowning.

"Yeah."

Julie bit back her initial comment, which was developing along the lines that he was smarter than any jock. Instead she asked, "Do you know what people who graduate with a degree in phys-ed do? What kind of jobs do they get?"

Pete shrugged. Silence, then, "In that book on biomechanics it said they can become trainers for athletes or pro teams, or physiotherapists or researchers figuring out how to help athletics get better."

Julie nodded. It was far from what she had ever envisioned for her son, but at least it appeared to be something he might be interested in. "You're truly interested in it?"

Pete thought for a moment, nodded and said, "Yeah, I think so."

He sounded far from convinced, but Julie pounced on the idea. "Then you better see about switching majors."

A professor is one who talks
in someone else's sleep.

—W. H. Auden, English poet, 1907-1973

April

"Research has shown that about half the speed of a pitch in base-ball is due to the pitcher's mechanics," the aged, elfin professor said as Pete sat at the back of the classroom nearest the door.

Pete let his eyes wander over toward a pretty brunette sitting two rows in front of him. He could just see the pleasing curve of her right breast straining the white cotton fabric of her Oxy T-shirt.

"The most important mechanical factor is the timing of maximum arm velocity. Now, you're wondering what that means?"

Pete glanced at the bespectacled, pale professor and thought, 'No, no one was wondering that, least of all me.' Pete had hoped he would learn something in biomechanics that would help him win some sports bets, but so far he had learned nothing of value.

"When a pitcher extends his elbow and internally rotates his shoulder, it is crucial to pitching speed," the prof explained, extending his frail left arm as if he was throwing a baseball. In his sixties, he looked like there was more of a chance that he would twist his arm off than throw a ball more than three feet. "How much the trunk stretches during the pitch is also crucially important."

"What determines the other half of pitching speed?" a diligent, muscular woman in the first row asked without raising her hand.

"Ah, yes, such things as how big a pitcher is and their strength, of course, directly affect the speed of the pitch; hence the tendency toward bigger and bigger pitchers in baseball."

Pete let out a sigh. How could even sports be made boring?

The day after Passover, Pete announced at dinner, "I dropped out."

Mentally, physically and emotionally exhausted, Julie couldn't believe what she'd heard. On top of long hours at the clinic, they had just sold their house and moved into a three-bedroom condo to help make her reduced income better meet their bills. "What?"

"I quit college today."

"You can't," Julie said, slamming her knife and fork down on the table, rattling the dishes. "Have you even thought about this or is it just another one of your rash decisions?"

"I have," Pete said, his voice devoid of emotion.

"You have got to get a degree, Pete."

"Why?"

"To get a decent job you have to have a college degree."

"There are jobs out there."

"Then find one," Julie snapped, losing patience. What had happened to Pete? Steroids, gambling, no interest in college, and now quitting? Had she raised him that poorly? It was on the tip of her tongue to say that it had been a monumental waste to put so much money into his college fund, but instead she said, "If you aren't going to school, you either have to get a job or move out. I'm not having you sitting around doing nothing all day."

"I found a job."

Julie stopped mid rant. "Doing what?"

"Coaching football to some kids at Veteran's Park for the city."

"Does it pay?"

"Of course it pays."

"How much?"

"Not much, but," Pete rushed to add before Julie could say anything, "I like it."

Envy eats nothing but its own heart.

—German proverb

Four years later, April

"I'm going for a jog," Adina announced, as she emerged from their Culver City condo's bedroom. She wore a black jogging suit with white stripes down the outside of each leg, which accented her long, slender legs. Even though her track scholarship to Arizona State had ended her second year when her times fell well behind those of her NCAA rivals—some of whom Pete suspected of steroid use or blood-doping—she had earned her bachelor's degree and even now kept running as if she was still in training. "Want to come?"

"I'm watching the draft," Pete said from the couch as he sucked down a diet cola, a biography of Mike Singletary lying open, face down beside him. The novel, *Huckleberry Finn*, sat on the end table by his elbow, a bookmark two-thirds of the way through its pages.

Adina asked, "Anyone we know?"

"Vikings took Joe Cain in the second round."

Adina stopped and watched the television from behind the sofa over Pete's shoulder. "Jayden?"

Pete fought to keep the envy out of his voice as he said, "Gonna freeze his tail off in Chicago as a Bear."

Just back from her honeymoon with Alan in Belize, Julie opened the mail. A white envelope held a golf scorecard and a piece of heavy white stationary folded in half. Frowning, she glanced at the scorecard. At the far right someone had circled the number 83 in pencil and underlined the figure three times with a black felt pen. She unfolded the stationary and read;

"Dear Dr. Stein,

I hope this finds you, since it took my grandson some doing to discover your home address. I wanted you to know that last week, at the age of 84, I shot an 83 at Riviera Country Club: besting my age.

Thank you for performing the surgery to remove my pituitary tumor a few years ago. If you had not, I would never have had the past few years of golf, the time with my family or the joys both have brought—and I never would have shot my age.

Sincerely and with greatest thanks, Tom Morris."

*Football players, like prostitutes, are in
the business of ruining their bodies for the
pleasure of strangers.*

—Merle Kessler, US writer, b. 1945

Seventeen years later, October

From the Minneapolis-St. Paul *StarTribune*:

Ex-Vike Linebacker
Joe Cain Dead at 39

Joe Cain, an ex-middle linebacker with the Minnesota Vikings, died yesterday of a stroke at his restaurant, The Spartan, in downtown Minneapolis.

At 6' 3" and 230 pounds, Cain was known during his career as an aggressive, dominating middle
linebacker.

"He was fierceness itself on the field," Jayden
Andrews, ex-linebacker for the Chicago Bears and
a high school teammate of Cain, said. "Those eyes
bore through you like a diamond drill."

In his first game as a starter, the seventh of his
rookie season with the Vikings, Cain recorded 10

tackles and forced a fumble. In his five-year career with the Vikings and Packers, he led each team in tackles every year until his final year. A series of injuries to his knees and back forced his early retirement.

After his playing days were over, Cain opened a restaurant in Minneapolis, his wife's hometown. As well as participating in various business ventures, he was active in many charities, including the United Way, DARE, Dads Against Drugs, and Athletes Against Steroids.

He is survived by his mother, Cheryl, brother, Daryn, sister, Sylvia, and his wife, Heather, and their three children, Sam, Vincent and Walter.

Julie added her latest rejection letter to her file, now held in three bulging file folders. Over the years, she had published two more short stories in obscure literary journals, but neither had led to any agent interest in one of her novels, let alone to an avalanche of publications.

As she ran her finger across the top of the thick rejection files, she wondered what would have happened if she had kept taking the drugs from her clinical trial: publications, fame, fortune and success or sickness, a stroke and death?

The list of drugs for her clinical trial flitted through her mind and then, unbidden, the evening she made her deal with Pete burst from her memory. She had made a deal, which he had kept. She wondered if he regretted it or if he thought it had saved his life. In either case, she had kept her word, too—at great cost.

She returned to her laptop and opened the file for the novel and outline that the agent had just rejected. She opened the list of agents she planned to send it to next. Keeping that file open on the left side of the screen to see where her dream would lead next, she started the laborious process of once again editing the novel's sample chapters.

When you look at where team sports are
going, the National Football league is
turning into organized warfare.

—Oren Lyons, Jr., National Lacrosse Hall
of Fame member, Faithkeeper of the Turtle
Clan, Seneca Nation of the Iroquois
Confederacy, b. 1930

Four years later, February

"Jayden's dead," Pete told Adina as she came home from work.

"Oh, no, I'm so sorry to hear that," she said, putting her bag
down on the narrow table in the entryway. With a compassionate
frown, she asked, "What happened?"

"Heart attack," Pete said, closing the black binder on the 670
defensive plays based on 66 different formations he had developed
for the team he coached at Windsor High School. "Last time we
talked, he mentioned he was having some problems with his heart.
The kids are at Mom's."

"Did he say it was serious?" she asked as she walked into the
living room.

"Said it wasn't anything to worry about, something about it being just the price of playing football."

"How's Janette taking it?"

"All tore up."

"How old was he?"

"Same as me, 43."

"What a waste," Adina said with a sad, slow shake of her head.

Pete frowned. "He had a great life. He played seven years for the Bears, and coached for a dozen more for the Cardinals, Patriots and Seahawks. He made millions. People stopped him for his autograph most everywhere he went. Quite a life."

"Dead at 43," Adina said, appalled. "Not even half a life." Seeing where his thoughts were taking him, she added in a harsh tone, "If you hadn't made that deal with your mom, you'd be dead, too."

"He got a Super Bowl ring with the Bears and another as a coach with the Patriots."

"So? Is that going to help Janette any?"

"The money he made will."

Adina let out a derisive snort. "I'm sure she'd rather have Jayden back than any amount of money."

Pete rose from the sofa and went into the kitchen where he poured himself a glass of orange juice. Adina followed, nodding in response to his questioning glance about whether she wanted a glass, too.

"He'll miss seeing his kids grow up, graduate high school, go to college, and start families of their own," Adina said, accepting the glass of juice from Pete. "He'll never hold his grandchildren and his grandchildren will never know him."

"I'm sure Janette will tell them stories about Jayden, like the time he intercepted a pass against the Packers in the final 20 seconds of a playoff game to take the Bears to the Super Bowl."

"There's more to life than just a game, Pete. There's being a husband and father, having a family and friends."

"Everyone can have a family; almost no one plays in the NFL, let alone in a Super Bowl."

"I guess you'd trade me and the kids for a chance to play a season in the NFL." Seeing the look on his face, she added with a dry laugh, "No, you'd trade us for a chance to play in a NFL game for a single play."

Sons are for fathers the twice-told tale.

—Victoria Secunda, *Women and Their Fathers,*
1992

April

Pete arrived home from coaching a spring practice camp Wednesday afternoon to cries of, "Daddy, daddy!"

His daughter, Juliana, raced toward him and enveloped him in a perfect tackle around the knees. At 3, she was already an all-star linebacker—at least against her father.

"Hi, Juliana, how are you?"

"Good, Daddy! I'm so happy you're home."

She clung to him like a limpet on an especially choice rock. His legs and knees ached, but he didn't shake her off. "I'm happy to be home, too, Chicklet."

"Hi, Dad," Tim, 7, called from the sofa, where he was playing a computer game.

"Where's your mom?"

"Downstairs doing laundry," Tim replied. He shut down the game and, grabbing a football off the sofa, asked, "Can we go to the park and play catch, Dad?"

"Maybe after dinner," Pete said, setting his bag on the hall table. He was debating whether to sit down with a novel, *Piece of Cake*, his mother had recommended and put ice on his knees. It sometimes helped, but invariably Adina and the kids cross-examined him about why he was icing them. How many times had he told them his knees, shoulders and back often hurt? For some reason they never believed him. "I'm beat. I got those books on sailing ships I promised to get for you from the library."

"Juliana wants to go to the park, too," Tim chided, ignoring the offered books.

"Please, Daddy, please," Juliana yelled, looking up at her father with her big, dark eyes and tilting her head to the side just as Adina did when she asked him to do something he didn't want to do.

"Why don't we read a book or something?" Pete felt all of his 44 years.

"Please, Dad," Tim begged, tossing the football at Pete, who caught it one-handed with long-practiced ease. "We never play football any more."

Pete looked down at the ball. His brow furrowed and his mood darkened. "Tim, how many times have I told you not to play with this ball?" The football had the Bears logo and the date and score of the game from which it came: Bears 24, Vikings 21. Jayden had sent it with a note to say he figured Pete would appreciate the game ball since Jayden's Bears beat Joe Cain's Vikes that blizzard-swept day at Soldier Field.

Tim shrank before his father's rebuke. Pete stalked over and set the precious ball on its wood stand on the bookshelf, which was otherwise crowded with Pete's novel collection, ranging from classics to recent bestsellers. Pete's hand rested on the ball as he stared at the Bear's logo and the cobweb of players' signatures in black and blue ink covering the rough surface. He spotted Jayden's scrawl; Jayden who had made a game-saving tackle and been awarded the game ball.

Turning from the ball and seeing his son's remorse, Pete said, his voice losing its edge, "Let's go for a swim instead. We can go to the park tomorrow. Juliana, you love swimming, don't you?" The pool would be a lot easier on his knees.

Juliana exploded, "Goodie, goodie, goodie, we're going swimming!"

Pete sat at Omar's garage on a white plastic lawnchair that had seen cleaner days. The chair was hard and uncomfortable, but it beat standing on the unforgiving blacktop with his wobbly knees while he waited for Omar to work some magic once again on Pete's ancient car. This time it was the alternator, but Pete knew that the real reason his 16-year-old car was in the shop again was, as Omar put it, because "She wheezes, rattles and creaks, just like the old woman she is."

"With two kids, a mortgage and bills that come in batches," Pete asked Omar, "How am I ever going to afford a new car on a high school coach's salary?"

Omar shrugged.

Pete sighed, rubbed his right knee and glanced over with a malevolent glare at his dented and dirty red sedan.

"At least I can have the kids wash it this weekend," he called to Omar.

"They'll love that," Omar said.

'So will I,' Pete thought as he opened Thomas Hardy's *Jude the Obscure*. It was one of his mom's recommendations.

After a few pages his attention was drawn to a black Mercedes sedan as it swung into the garage's oil-spotted lot. Pete watched the immaculate German car stop without a sound, ruefully recalling the squeaks that his car emitted every time it stopped. New brakes would have to wait.

A slight, dark-haired man with stylish, silver-framed sunglasses and dressed in khakis and a golf shirt slid out of the Mercedes. He swung the door closed without a sound and strode over toward Omar, who, wiping his hands on a greasy rag, came out of one of the service bays to meet him. Pete watched the new customer, thinking that he knew the man, but was unable to place him. The man seemed to be Pete's age, but Pete was far from certain. He looked younger than Pete, but carried himself as if he was older or at least held great authority and a vast reservoir of confidence.

Pete's eyes swung back to the Mercedes as a pretty, petite woman slid out of the passenger side. She wore tight blue jeans that accented her hips and a white blouse that hinted at a nice chest. Her dark brown hair was shoulder length and, even Pete could tell, had been cut by someone who knew what they were doing. The woman's face was open and friendly with large, dark eyes and a mouth that turned up at either end, as if in a perpetual smile. She looked like the sort of woman who had a great body, but felt no need to show it.

As Pete admired her, the rear doors opened and two kids scrambled out: a dark-haired, energetic boy and a curly-haired, smiling girl. They were about the same age as Pete's kids.

As Pete watched, the man finished talking to Omar, walked back to the woman and the children, and spoke with them. Whatever was said, the woman took charge of the kids and headed toward the corner. From where the kids were looking, Pete guessed they were headed to the mini-market across the street.

Pete turned back to his novel.

Having surveyed the garage's lot, the man with the Mercedes sauntered over to where Pete sat. He hesitated as he glanced down at one of the other dirty, white, plastic chairs.

"It's clean, even if it doesn't look it," Pete said. He had tested his chair before sitting down and found that although the chairs looked grimy, the dirt was so imbedded that it didn't come off on your hand or your clothes.

"Thanks," the man said and sat down.

Pete rubbed his right knee. Now from up close, Pete realized who it was. "Mike Lowe," he exclaimed, surprised and happy that he had recognized his old schoolmate.

Mike turned and, peering at Pete, said as a grin spread across his face, "Pete Tomlinson."

They shook hands.

"Live around here?" Pete asked.

"Just down the coast. We were on our way up to our cabin in Big Bear to do some mountain biking when my wife's car started vibrating on the freeway. Thought it might be a strut, so I wanted to have it checked out."

"Where do you live?"

"Manhattan Beach."

Pete nodded. Manhattan Beach was nice.

"You?"

"Culver City," Pete said. Not quite as nice as Manhattan Beach. "I haven't seen you in years. Did you ever make it to the Ivy League?"

"Well, sort of," Mike replied, grinning. "MIT."

"Isn't that Ivy League?" If they didn't have a big-name football program, what Pete knew about colleges could fit on a postage stamp.

"No, it's not, but it was better for engineering."

Pete recalled that Mike had wanted to be an engineer in high school. "I coach football over at Windsor High," Pete offered, not knowing why he said it.

"You were always into football," Mike commented, his eyes wandering over to a pretty redhead who was filling up her silver Lexus at a pump.

"What do you do for a living?"

Mike pulled his dark brown eyes back from admiring the redhead. "I'm a partner at Larson and Lee."

Pete's eyes narrowed. "Aren't they building the new wing on Windsor High?" There was a sign at his school.

"I believe so. It's one of our smaller projects, so I'm not involved with it."

"What do you do?"

"Office buildings, malls and high-rise condominiums mostly."

Pete nodded. "What's your wife do?"

"Makes sure the kids don't burn down the house."

Pete wished Adina could stay home, but it was out of the question if they wanted to live anywhere on the west side of Los Angeles. It was just too expensive for one income unless, Pete thought glancing at Mike, you were a partner in a civil engineering firm.

Mike asked, "You?"

"I married Adina Gebreyohannes," Pete said, grinning at the thought of the pretty girl he had convinced to marry him.

"She ran track, didn't she?" Mike said, frowning as he searched his memory.

"Right the first time."

"I knew most of the members of the track team, but not her."

Pete thought, 'That's because she didn't take steroids,' but didn't say it.

Omar sauntered over, his long legs covering the distance quickly as he gestured to Mike, who rose, bid Pete goodbye and walked over to find out whether he and his family would make it mountain biking today.

Pete had read a few more pages of the tragedy of Jude Fawley when Mike's pretty wife and cute kids arrived back from the store, sodas and snacks in their hands. Pete sighed, leaned back in the sun and watched Mike and his family stroll down the street window shopping while they waited for their car.

"Know him?" Omar asked as he slouched beside Pete, an oil-stained cigarette drooping from the corner of his mouth.

"Went to high school together," Pete said, glancing over at his old car.

"She's ready," Omar replied to Pete's unspoken question. "Your friend's doing well."

"An upstart," Pete agreed with a thin smile.

Omar frowned. "Is that an American thing?"

"It's someone who's done far better than their parents."

"My father owned a 50,000-hectare ranchero in Argentina," Omar said. "Now I own this." He gestured back at his two-bay garage.

"What happened to the ranch?"

"My older brother got it; all 50,000 hectares, 4,000 head of cattle, and a nice life as the *jefe* of a couple of dozen *vaqueros*."

"You and I are what my grandfather called 'downstarts,'" Pete said with a chuckle. "We did worse than our parents."

"You must do pretty good," Omar said, waving his cigarette in the air with his oil- and grease-stained hand.

"Not so much; college and the pros is where the real money is."

Pete had applied several times to be a college assistant coach with the goal of moving up to become a head coach. Without any collegiate playing experience, let alone any time in the pros, it had proved impossible to even get an interview.

"At least we're doing what we love to do," Omar said with a broad grin. "You, football and me, cars."

Pete smiled. "I used to love to play."

"Bet the girls loved you," Omar said with a leering grin.

Pete laughed. "A freshman girl once offered to sleep with me, no strings attached. Wanted to be able to say she'd bedded a football player."

"How was it?"

"I had a girlfriend."

"Too bad. Would have made a better story if you'd said yes. Play football any more?"

Pete shook his head. "By the time I was 20, I had bad knees, a bad back, and enough aches and pains for a lifetime."

"At least you coach football."

"Keeps me in the game," Pete agreed, although the sadness and longing in his voice came through in his words. What if he had never made that deal with his mom? Would he have played in the NFL like Jayden and Joe Cain, signing autographs, making millions, driving a Mercedes with a pretty wife beside him? Or would he be dead? Either way, it was done now. He couldn't go back. No amount of steroids could fix his knees and back enough to enable him to play in a high school game, let alone college or the pros. Worse, he thought with sorrow, he was too old. Some dreams had time limits.

Pete rose and, slipping a gold-embossed leather bookmark from the LA County Library into his novel, walked with Omar over toward the office to settle his account. Every step he took he remembered a game, a play or a tackle from his high school days. They were burned into his mind with a clarity that surpassed that of any of the other memories he carried.

As Pete walked past, he admired Mike's new Mercedes and wondered. Maybe his mom had been right to push him toward college. Was it too late? There had to be more to life, more he could do.

As they stepped into the office, struck by a sudden impulse, Pete asked Omar, "What do you think about the name, The Pete Tomlinson Football Schools?"

Sic transit gloria mundi

—Latin Proverb
"Thus passes the glory of the world"
or
"All glory is fleeting"

Ten years later, February

Julie sat on the sofa to start writing a new book. Her fingers throbbed with arthritis. Her wrist where she had broke it more than 30 years before ached with a dull, cold pain; it often did now when the temperature fell. Glancing at herself in the mirror above the fireplace of the home she had shared with Alan until six months ago, she saw that she was still slim and straight-backed, but her hair had turned silver and her face betrayed her years in countless wrinkles around the eyes, mouth and neck. Her skin had taken on a translucent appearance. Looking down at her hands, she saw the gnarled, wrinkled hands of a woman in her seventies. Worse, her memory was slipping; not the forgetfulness that everyone has for a name, a date or where they left their car keys, but the terrifying lack of memory for what car keys are for. Such memory deficits are an early symptom of Alzheimer's disease. Time was running out.

Putting the aches, pains and worries aside, she debated whether what she planned to write should be a novel or a memoir. She quickly decided that decision could wait. Once she had written a

few pages, she would know which form would seem right. She
started tapping the keys on her laptop:

"I dreamed of being the greatest writer ever and for two months
I was. For such a brief time, I could write like Twain, Hemingway
or even Shakespeare, and not the Shakespeare of his lesser known
works. Not like when he wrote *Titus Andronicus*, which is so inferior
his supporters claim the bard never even wrote it. For that brief
time, I could write as sweetly as the sweet swan of Avon at his
sweetest when he penned the immortal *Lear*, *Hamlet* and *Macbeth*.

"If only I had written my story then, it would have been great.
I would have been great. If only. Now I struggle to find the right
words, belaboring every word, phrase and sentence. It is as painful
as childbirth or a broken wrist.

"Right words or not, I must try to tell my story or it will gnaw at
me, reminding me of my dream and how far my outstretched fingers are from touching it. Robert Browning wrote, 'Ah, but a man's
reach should exceed his grasp, or what's a heaven for?' Once I not
only touched my dream, but grasped it and held it tight with both
hands, but now my dream—my heaven—is far beyond my reach.
Having tasted it, felt it, breathed the air of my private heaven, I
have learned to live with the fact that I may never again touch it, let
alone grasp it. I fear that the brief time when I lived my dream is
gone, and gone forever; such is my private hell. Worse, I share that
hell with my son.

"I gave up my dream for my son and he gave up his dream for
me. Now that we know what abandoning our dreams has cost, I
wonder how long we would hesitate to surrender our dreams now
or if we would give them up at all for anything or anyone—even
for each other.

"Whatever the answer, what is done, is done. Few things about
the past can be changed and those that can be changed often can
only be changed when it is too late. I know it is too late for my son,
but maybe it is not too late for me.

"This is our story."

The only yardstick for success our society has is being a champion. No one remembers anything else.

—John Madden, US football player and coach, b. 1936

May

"Mom," Pete called as he let himself into her house with his key.

Alan had passed away from liver disease just nine months before. The funeral at Arlington had been hard on his mom, but Lieutenant General Alan McGhee had wanted the full military sendoff with The Old Guard performing honor guard duties, a full-dress bugler playing Taps, and the crack of rifles in salute. Compounding his mother's grief, Pete's aunt had died of breast cancer just six months ago.

With understandable cause, Pete's mom had been depressed in the fall, although she had markedly improved in the winter and spring. She had even stopped smoking, again. But even with an improved mental outlook, she had rarely wanted to come over to Pete's house, let alone have him visit her. She always said she was busy. Tonight, Pete wanted to get her out of the house, willing or not. They were going out to dinner at Asia de Cuba, his mom's favorite.

"Mom," he called again.

At 54, Pete was still fit, even if he did sport a paunch. He wore a sweatshirt with "Pete Tomlinson Football Schools" emblazoned across the chest. On the back it proclaimed, "Twenty-five Graduates in the NFL and Counting!"

Pete walked through the modern kitchen, stopping to glance at a bookcase in the short hall that led to the living room. He had read most of the novels on the shelves, but spotted a couple he would have to ask to borrow. He chuckled at the thought that as a teenager he had never even glanced at the books on his mom's bookcase. Now he had more bookshelves than she did.

"Mom," he called again, frowning as he saw her lying on the sofa. Something was wrong. A sheaf of papers had fluttered off her lap onto the floor. More striking was the fact that her face and body were too relaxed: no one ever looked that relaxed, even in the deepest sleep. The muscles of her face had a looseness that was inhuman.

As he stepped toward her, the brutal, foul smell hit him. For an instant he thought he was going to vomit. Inhaling rapid, short breaths, he approached her and, touching a hand to her cheek, confirmed what he feared. She was cold.

After calling 9-1-1, he went into the bathroom to get a facecloth to wipe the tears from his face before the paramedics arrived. His head ached from crying. He had not even realized the tears had been flowing until he noticed that his face was wet.

After drying his face with a white towel, he opened the medicine cabinet to see if there was aspirin for his headache. He stopped. He stared at the row of prescription bottles on the glass shelves. Scanning the names, he was jolted back into the past: they were the drugs from the Alzheimer's clinical trial his mom had conducted so many years before. He would never forget the names he had seen as he had pounded the pills in piles with his steroids into powder with a hammer.

Pete slammed the cabinet door closed in a rage. The glass face shattered. Jagged pieces tinkled as they struck the tile floor.

He stalked back into the living room and yelled at his mother, "How could you?"

He slumped into a swivel chair near his mom, cradling his head with his hands. He reached over and scooped up the papers that had slipped to the floor. Without meaning to, he began to read. It was a novel. After a few pages, even through his grief, pain and anguish, he knew that the opening was good, even great.

He swore and glared over at his dead mother.

Shaking his head, on impulse he stalked over to the fireplace and, igniting the gas, thrust the manuscript pages one by one into the fire until they were all incinerated.

Just as he finished his vengeful chore, the doorbell rang; the paramedics, not that they could do any good now.

He rose, tears streaming down his face. As he walked past his mother's body, he said, "We had a deal."

Forgiveness is the final form of love.

—Reinhold Niebuhr, US theologian,
1892-1971

Pete wandered into his mom's home office and sat at the computer. Adina and the kids were in the kitchen sorting everything into piles for Goodwill, the food bank, a garage sale or to be taken home.

Pete skimmed through the files on his mom's computer. He stopped at one dated the day she died. He opened the Word file captioned "Novel 36" and began to read.

"Pete, Pete," Adina called, placing a hand on his shoulder.

Pete jumped and looked up.

"What are you reading?" Adina asked, peering over his shoulder at the screen. "You didn't hear me calling?"

"Something Mom wrote." He had read 74 pages. He wiped his wet eyes as if he had something in them.

"It's late. Should we head home for dinner?"

Pete nodded.

Adina left to tell the kids. It was later than Pete had thought. Even so, he sat and stared at the text before him. Moments later as he heard Adina telling the kids to get ready to go, he closed the file. His gaze fell on a file called, Agents. He considered for a moment, sighed and, calling out that he'd be a few more minutes, clicked on the agent file.

"It's the finest piece of writing I've read since she sent us those chapters years ago," agent Charles Wood-Byrd told Jonathan Sharpe, CEO and Publisher of Kira House Press. "Do you recall?"

"How couldn't I? One of the finest beginnings of a novel I've ever read, but it most certainly didn't follow through in terms of quality," Jonathan observed, stretching back in the plush armchair across from Charles' ornate, but battered desk. Jonathan blew on his tea to cool it.

"Truth be told, I was reluctant to read it, but I started late in the day and before I knew it, I had read the entire thing," Charles said with chagrin. "I failed to arrive home until 5 in the morning. Virginia was mad as hell, wondering where on God's green earth I'd been. Apparently I failed to hear my telephone ringing."

"Do you represent her this time?" Jonathan asked with a wry grin as he sipped his steaming tea from a white mug in the cramped office, cluttered with manuscripts, books and framed photographs of the agent with a writer's convention worth of top authors.

"I'm saddened to say that she recently passed on."

"How'd you get the manuscript then?"

"Her son sent it with a kind note saying he would be much in my debt if I would represent his mother's literary estate, namely this novel."

"You think it's good?"

"It's a masterpiece.

About the Author

The author of two non-fiction books, K. Scot Macdonald has also contributed to two edited volumes and to *The Writers' Journal*. He lives in California with his wife, daughter, and two Scottish terriers. To find out more about him, visit KScotMacdonald.com.

About Kerrera House Press

Kerrera House Press is an independent press dedicated to producing the books you keep. Visit us at KerreraHousePress.com.

Reader Resources

For a reader's guide, character bios and more about the story and writing of *The Shakespeare Drug*, please visit KerreraHousePress.com.

www.ingramcontent.com/pod-product-compliance
Lightning Source LLC
Chambersburg PA
CBHW031552240626
47153CB00002B/476

* 9 7 8 0 9 8 5 9 6 5 0 0 6 *